Heart Disease
No More!

*Make Peace with Your Heart
and Heal Yourself*

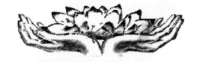

Your Health is in Your Hands

For Reasons of Legality

The author of this book, Andreas Moritz, does not advocate the use of any particular form of health care but believes that the facts, figures, and knowledge presented herein should be available to every person concerned with improving his or her state of health. Although the author has attempted to give a profound understanding of the topics discussed and to ensure accuracy and completeness of any information that originates from any other source than his own, he and the publisher assume no responsibility for errors, inaccuracies, omissions, or any inconsistency herein. Any slights of people or organizations are unintentional. This book is not intended to replace the advice and treatment of a physician who specializes in the treatment of diseases. Any use of the information set forth herein is entirely at the reader's discretion. The author and publisher are not responsible for any adverse effects or consequences resulting from the use of any of the preparations or procedures described in this book. The statements made herein are for educational and theoretical purposes only and are mainly based upon Andreas Moritz's own opinion and theories. You should always consult with a health care practitioner before taking any dietary, nutritional, herbal or homeopathic supplement, or beginning or stopping any therapy. The author is not intending to provide any medical advice, or offer a substitute thereof, and make no warranty, expressed or implied, with respect to any product, device or therapy, whatsoever. Except as otherwise noted, no statement in this book has been reviewed or approved by the United States Food & Drug Administration or the Federal Trade Commission. Readers should use their own judgment or consult a holistic medical expert or their personal physicians for specific applications to their individual problems.

ISBN: 0-9767944-5-4

Published by Ener-Chi Wellness Press (Ener-chi.com), U.S.A.
Excerpted from *Timeless Secrets of Health & Rejuvenation*, Aug. 2005
Cover Design/Artwork (Ener-chi Art for the Heart, Oil on Canvas):
 By Andreas Moritz

. . .

Your heart is the most precious and life-giving organ you have. Moment by moment, day after day and year after year, your heart takes you through life without faltering or missing a beat. However, your heart requires good care, happiness, and proper sustenance to pump the right amount of blood through the body and allow its trillions of cells to breathe and be nourished. Heart disease shows you have neglected your heart. By taking care of your heart, your heart will take care of you for the rest of your life.

Andreas Moritz

. . .

Also by Andreas Moritz

. . .

**The Amazing Liver
& Gallbladder Flush**

**Timeless Secrets of
Health & Rejuvenation**

Lifting the Veil of Duality

Cancer Is Not A Disease (New)

It's Time to Come Alive

The Art of Self Healing
(Mid-2006)

Simple Steps to Total Health
(Mid-2006)

Sacred Santémony

Ener-Chi Art

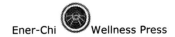

Ener-Chi   Wellness Press

Table of Contents

Heart Disease No More

Disease – Symptom Of A Sick Body   **1**

The Beginning Stages Of Heart Disease   3

Major Contributing Factors   5

Meat Consumption And Heart Disease   7

Your Body Can Store Protein!   9

Protein Storage – A Time Bomb   17

The Revealing Role Of Homocysteine   20

C-Reactive Protein Reveals The Truth   22

How Heart Attacks Really Occur   25

Heart Attacks Can Occur In A Number Of Ways: 26

New Studies Question Value Of Opening Arteries   27

Risk Indications Of A Heart Attack   **33**

1.   Thickening Of Blood As Measured By   35
      Hemocrit (Packed Cell Volume)

2.   Eating Too Much Animal Protein   37

3.   Cigarette Smoking   38

4.   Constitutional (Genetic) Disposition   39
      Towards Reduced Protein Breakdown

5.   Women During And After Menopause   40

6.   Not Eating Enough Fruit And Vegetables; 41
      Smoking; Lack Of Exercise

7.   Kidney Disease   46

8.   Antibiotics And Other Synthetic Drugs   49

Ending The Cholesterol - Heart Disease   54
Myth
Cholesterol – Not The Culprit After All   50

Death in Trans Fatty Acids   56

Healthy Today – Sick Tomorrow   60

What Statins May Do To You!   65

But Doesn't Aspirin Protect Against Heart 73
Disease?

Dangers Of Low Cholesterol   75

Cholesterol – Your Life And Blood 80

When Cholesterol Signals SOS 84

Balancing Cholesterol Levels Naturally 89

Overcoming Heart Disease – Two Encouraging 92
Testimonies

Non-Dietary Causes Of Heart Disease 96

Lack Of Social Support System 96

Greatest Risk Factors: 98
Job Satisfaction And Happiness Rating

Your Need To Love 101

The Power of A Loving Spouse 103

The Healing Power Of "Loving Touch" 105

Conclusion 109

Useful Tips to Reverse Heart Disease 111

About The Author 113

Other Books, Products And Services 116
By The Author

Heart Disease No More!

Symptom of a Sick Body

L ess than 100 years ago heart disease was an extremely rare disease. Today, it kills more people in the developed world than all other causes of death taken together (with the exception of doctor-caused, iatrogenic, diseases[1]). According to the *New England Journal of Medicine*, sudden cardiac arrest claims 350,000 to 450,000 lives per year in the United States (over 1,000 per day) and is responsible for more than half of all deaths that are due to cardiovascular disease. Over 860,000 Americans suffer a heart attack each year. In the U.S., there are 7.8 million heart attack survivors (as per year 2004). Direct (medical costs) and indirect (lost productivity) costs related to coronary heart disease were about $133 billion in 2004. A recent study concludes that 85% of people over 50 already have artery blockages… and 71% of people over 40!

Although the ability to recognize patients who are at high risk for cardiac arrest has greatly improved over the past 20 years, 90 percent of cases of sudden death from cardiac

---

[1] See Chapter 14 of *Timeless Secrets of Health & Rejuvenation*

1

causes occur in patients without identified risk factors. It is known that the majority of cases of sudden death from cardiac causes involve patients with preexisting coronary heart disease. Yet cardiac arrest is the first manifestation of this underlying problem in 50 percent of patients.

The most common underlying cause of sudden cardiac arrest is a heart attack which causes irregular heart rhythm and subsequent stoppage of the heart. In several industrialized nations, mortality rates from heart attacks have slightly decreased due to a generation of breakthroughs in heart care. These include new medicines, the bypass operations, and the angioplasties. Now many of the "beneficiaries" of this kind of heart care are living with unexpected, often devastating consequences: Their damaged hearts still beat, but not strong enough to enjoy a decent quality of life. Many wish they had died swiftly than suffering a slow and torturous death.

The unintended result of better cardiac care is an unprecedented increase in a chronic, debilitating disease called *chronic heart failure*, which we could easily call an epidemic. Heart failure is described as a *gradual* ebbing of the heart's power to pump blood and supply the body with oxygen. "Heart failure is a product of our success in dealing with heart disease and hypertension," said Dr. Michael Bristow of the

University of Colorado. Treating the symptoms of heart disease and hypertension rather than their causes has lead to more hardship and suffering than anticipated. It is the call of our time to take a more holistic look at the causes of this greatest killer disease in the modern world and to apply natural methods to restore heart functions swiftly and permanently, without side effects.

The Beginning Stages of Heart Disease

Our cardiovascular system is composed of a central pumping device – the heart muscles – and a blood vessel pipeline, consisting of arteries, veins and capillaries. The heart muscles pump blood through the blood vessel system to deliver oxygen and nutrients to all parts of the body. The blood vessel system is over 60,000 miles long and has a surface of more than half an acre. The 60 – 100 trillion cells in the body depend on the frictionless flow of blood through this vast network of channels.

The tiny blood capillaries, which have the thickness of one tenth of a human hair, are of particular importance to the body. Unlike the arteries, capillaries permit oxygen, water, and nutrients to pass through their thin walls in order to bring nourishment to the surrounding tissues. At the same time, they have to allow certain cellular waste to return to the blood so that it can be excreted from the body. If the capillary network becomes congested for reasons explained below, the heart has to pump the blood with greater pressure to reach all the different parts of the body. This considerably increases the heart's workload and makes its muscles tense and tired. In due time, the exertion of the heart leads to stress and fatigue and impairs all major functions in the body.

Since the blood capillaries are also responsible for nourishing the muscle cells of the arteries, a reduced supply of oxygen, water, and nutrients will gradually injure and destroy arteries. To counteract this form of involuntary self-destruction, the body responds with inflammation. The inflammation response, which is often mistaken for and treated as a disease, is actually one of the body's best methods to increase the blood supply and deliver vital nutrients to promote growth of new cells and repair damaged connective tissue. However, continuous inflammatory responses eventually generate sizable lesions in the arteries, which, in turn, lead to the development of atherosclerotic deposits. Hardening of arteries (atherosclerosis) is commonly believed to be the main cause of heart disease, although this is, as new studies have shown, not entirely true.

Major Contributing Factors

Most heart disease patients and their doctors assume that heart attacks are triggered by the clogging of the heart arteries[2], which according to that assumption, destroys millions of heart cells. Similarly, strokes are thought to be caused by the clogging of the brain arteries, which causes the death of millions of brain cells. Since brain cells coordinate the activities and movements of every part of the body, their death can lead to partial or complete paralysis and death. A stroke is considered merely a consequence of advanced atherosclerosis.

The brain arteries are located in close proximity to the heart. The blood pressure in both the brain and heart arteries is relatively higher than in those arteries located in other parts of the body, hence the difference of blood pressure in the different arteries of the circulatory system. If turbulence and congestion occur in the branching areas of the arteries, the blood pressure begins to rise. This particularly stresses the coronary, carotid (neck), and cerebral (brain) arteries to the point

---

[2] As we will see, this assumption is not entirely correct.

5

of damage. Damage occurs first in those blood vessels that are already weakened by internal congestion and nutrient deficiencies. This makes high blood pressure a major risk factor for strokes and heart disease.

Lowering an elevated blood pressure through medication, however, does not serve as a solution, but as a mere postponement and further aggravation of the problem. Moreover, as recent research has shown, it can lead to chronic heart failure. Without removing the root cause(s) of elevated blood pressure the standard treatment for hypertension can cause severe cellular dehydration and sharply reduce the blood's capacity to deliver oxygen to the heart muscles and remove toxic waste from the cells and tissues of the body. All this further increases the risk of heart disease and many other health problems, including kidney and liver disorders.

Countries in the Western Hemisphere are heading the global list of heart disease. For many years, now, doctors have blamed the wrong type of food, overeating, too little exercise, smoking, and stress as the major risk factors. Latest research has added a few more, such as free radicals, pollution, poor circulation, certain drugs and chemicals, and a decreased ability of the blood to digest protein, which may lead to the formation of blood clots. When the proteolytic enzymes bromelain, trypsin, and chymotrypsin are no longer sufficiently available to help break down the blood clots, heart attacks, phlebitis, and stokes are the most likely consequences.

The greatest physical cause of coronary heart disease, however, is overeating of animal proteins. When stored in the body, protein becomes one of the greatest risk factors for heart disease and most other diseases as well. One of the latest markers of arterial damage and inflammation now believed to be the main reason behind blood clots triggering a heart attack is the protein *homocysteine.* High concentrations of homocysteine are found in meat.

Meat Consumption and Heart Disease

To illustrate the development of heart disease from virtual non-existence to being the biggest killer disease, I have used statistical trends describing disease development in Germany – a typical, modern industrialized nation. In the year 1800, meat consumption in Germany was about 13 kg (28 pounds) per person per year. One hundred years later, meat consumption was nearly three times as high, at 38 kg per person per year. By 1979, it had reached 94.2 kg, which is an increase of 725 percent in less than 180 years. These figures do not include fats. During the period of 1946-1978, meat consumption in Germany increased by 90% and heart attacks rose by 20 times. During the same period, fat consumption remained the same, whereas consumption of cereals and potatoes, which are major suppliers of vegetable protein, decreased by 45%. Therefore, fats and carbohydrates, as well as vegetable proteins, cannot be considered to be causes of coronary heart disease. This leaves meat as the main factor responsible for the dramatic upsurge of this degenerative blood vessel disease.

In consideration of the fact that at least 50 percent of the German population is overweight and most overweight people eat much more meat than those with normal weight do, meat consumption among the overweight must have at least quadrupled in the 33 years after World War II. Being overweight is considered to be a major risk for high blood pressure and heart disease.

According to statistics published by the World Health Organization (WHO) in 1978, the yearly increases of heart attacks in Western European countries were accompanied by a continuous yearly increase in meat consumption by as much as 4kg per person. This practically means that eating habits after

World War II have shifted from a healthy mixed diet to one excessive in animal protein, but poor in carbohydrates such as fruits, vegetables and grains. According to the WHO, fat consumption remained virtually unchanged. Heart attacks and atherosclerosis began to increase dramatically in Germany and in Western industrialized nations soon after the war; today they cause over 50 percent of all deaths.

Although fat consumption among vegetarians is not less than among meat eaters, the vegetarians have the lowest death rates from heart disease. The *Journal of the American Medical Association* reported that a vegetarian diet could prevent 97% of all coronary occlusions. The incredibly popular high protein, low carbohydrate *Atkins Diet* and *South Beach Diet* have the unfortunate side effect of starving a person by clogging up his capillary and artery walls with excessive proteins, and by greatly limiting his fuel intake (carbohydrates). This can certainly make a person lose weight, but not without also damaging his kidneys, liver, and heart. Both the late Dr. Atkins, a heart disease and obesity victim, and former U.S. President Bill Clinton, a keen follower of the South Beach Diet and recipient of a quadruple bypass, suffered the consequences of the high protein diet (for

9

details, see section below). Millions of Americans are following in their footsteps.

The reason for the virtual absence of coronary heart disease among vegetarians is their low intake or complete absence of animal protein. Fat consumption is, therefore, only an accomplice of the disease, but not its cause. The constantly recycled mass hysteria that believes fat, which is generally associated with cholesterol, to be the main dietary culprit of heart disease, is completely unfounded, outdated, and has no scientific basis.

Your Body Can Store Protein!

Meat and meat products have five to ten times the concentration of protein than found in plant protein foods. It is, therefore, easily possible to overeat animal protein, but it is hardly possible to overeat vegetable protein because a normal digestive system does not have the ability to process 5-10 times more food than is normal for the body. It is common knowledge that the body is able to store unused sugar and other carbohydrates in the form of fat, but it lesser known that it also has a large storage capacity for protein. The body's protein stores are the *connective tissues* (the fluids between the capillaries and the cells) and the

10

basal or *basement membranes*, which hold together and support the cells of the blood capillaries and arteries (see illustration 1). When these protein stores are filled to their full storage capacity, the organs and arteries that are supplied by these protein-congested capillaries begin to starve of oxygen and nutrients, and suffocate in their own metabolic waste products. The resulting toxicity crisis prompts an inflammatory process by the body, which is necessary to increase blood flow and make nutrients available for growth of new cells and repair of damaged connective tissue. Repeated bouts of inflammation in the artery walls can involve bleeding and subsequent formation of blood clots. Blood clots are the number one cause of heart attacks (see illustrations 2a/b) and strokes. As a measure of first aid and to avert constantly occurring potential heart attacks or strokes, the body attempts to contain the bleeding wounds. It does this by dispatching the glue-like *lipoprotein*, LP5, into the blood. LP5 attaches itself to the open wounds, thereby sealing them. To promote wounds healing and prevent them from repeated bleeding, the sticky LP5 catches the relatively large lipoprotein molecules, such as LDL and VLDL cholesterol molecules, and builds them into the artery walls. The resulting protective "bandage" saves the person's life, at least for a while. If this survival mechanism

11

occurs in the coronary arteries, it is called *hardening of arteries* or *coronary heart disease.*

A person who eats too many simple carbohydrate foods such as sugar, bread and pasta, or fats in a particular meal may have elevated concentrations of sugar, fats, and the cholesterol-containing *lipoproteins* in his blood. However, blood tests also show that if he overeats protein foods, his blood will contain higher concentrations of protein. Nutritional science assumes[3] that protein is completely burned during the digestive process. Whatever protein the body cells don't use or need, so goes the argument, continues to circulate in the blood until it is broken down by liver enzymes and excreted as urea.

A major problem arises when a person does not have enough of these enzymes to remove the excessive protein from the blood stream. The liver of Kapha and Pitta types, for example, who naturally require only very few proteins to sustain themselves, has a limited capacity to break down food proteins. If liver bile ducts are congested with stones, this also greatly diminishes this important liver function. The same applies to people who regularly eat too many proteins. In any case, the extra

---

[3] There is no scientific research to support this assumption

proteins that are not broken down and eliminated through the liver route, are absorbed by the connective tissue under the skin (which is the least harmful), and the intercellular connective tissue of the organs (which can be very harmful). If there is a continuous, regular supply of large amounts of food protein, the intercellular connective tissue and basal membranes of the capillaries start filling up with the protein and begin to thicken. Unless protein intake is discontinued, the capillary cells become damaged. The body responds with inflammation to help destruct and remove damaged or dead cells. This inflammatory process, though, has side-effects. It forms the beginning stage of diet-caused atherosclerosis.

By contrast, as it was first discovered in 1955, people who live on a protein-free diet for a certain length of time do not produce urea after their first protein meals. This means that their connective tissues contain no abnormal amounts of protein. This applies to all vegetarians whose only source of protein is of purely vegetarian origin, such as in grains, legumes, nuts, seeds, etc. Vegetarians hardly ever develop a surplus of protein in the connective tissues and blood vessel walls, and are, therefore, not at risk of developing atherosclerotic deposits. This has been confirmed by the American Medical Association.

It is a commonly accepted medical theory that all unused calories, whether they occur in the form of carbohydrates, fat, or protein, are converted into fat and deposited in the body's fat cells. This would make fat to be the only storage molecule responsible for obesity and related illnesses, including coronary heart disease and Type 2 diabetes[4]. Yet there is overwhelming evidence to show that stored fat alone cannot be held responsible for causing coronary heart disease. The only other substance that the body can store in large amounts is protein; much of it ends up in the blood vessel walls.

In addition to breaking down proteins in the liver and storing proteins in the blood vessel walls, the body employs another tactic to get rid of this dangerous culprit. A well-trained athlete can utilize no more than 40 grams of protein per day. The average American eats up 200 grams per day. Whatever proteins cannot be stored, which easily happens by regularly eating more than 30-40 grams of protein each day, the body converts into nitric, sulfuric and phosphoric acids. The kidneys try to eliminate some of the strong acids (similar to the ones found in your car battery). To do so, they have to attach a basic mineral to every acid

---

[4] See *Reversing Diabetes* or Chapter 11 of Timeless Secrets of Health & Rejuvenation

molecule, As a result, sodium, potassium, magnesium (the main basic minerals) and all the rest become depleted as well. All this sets your body up for an incidence of *acidosis*, which is another name for toxicity crisis. Heart disease is a typical symptom of chronic acidosis.

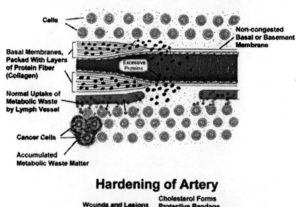

Illustration 1:
Congestion of Blood Vessel Walls
with Excessive Protein

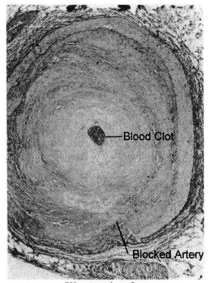

Illustration 2a:
Blood clot that caused heart attack
in a 54-year old man

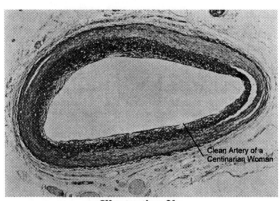

Illustration 2b:
Healthy, clear artery of a 100-year old woman

16

Protein Storage – A Time Bomb

Obese people have both high concentrations of fats and excessive amounts of protein in the blood. The blood's tendency towards clotting, which is considered to be the greatest risk for suffering a heart attack or stroke, stems almost exclusively from the saturation of the blood with proteins (also smoking increases blood protein concentrations, as shown below). Natural fats (except the unnatural trans fatty acids as found in hydrogenated vegetable oils and margarine), on the other hand, have *no* blood-clotting ability. In their attempt to avert a heart attack, the capillary cells absorb the excessive protein, convert it into *collagen-fiber,* and store it in their basement membranes. Although this emergency response has a blood-thinning and, therefore, life-saving effect, it also makes the blood walls thicker and more vulnerable to injury.

Examinations of connective tissue in obese people have proved that it contains not only plump fat cells, but also large amounts of dense collagen-fiber. Collagen is 100 percent pure protein. Building more collagen-fiber than necessary is one of the main emergency measures the body takes to deal with dangerously high protein concentrations in the blood. By removing the protein from the blood and thereby putting it out of circulation, the blood becomes thin and the crisis is avoided. However, the situation changes drastically when the body's protein stores are all filled up to capacity, and protein consumption continues. In such a situation, the blood becomes and remains saturated with protein. Hence, the blood begins to permanently thicken and develop a tendency towards clotting. Unless the afflicted person takes aspirin, which has a blood thinning effect, a stroke or a heart attack may occur. Yet in the long term, the drug not only fails to prevent such an incidence, but actually strongly encourages it. There is a heightened risk of deadly uncontrolled bleeding that comes with regular or excessive aspirin use. In addition, once aspirin treatment discontinues, the risk of suffering a heart attack is greatly increased. [**Warning:** If you are suffering from macular degeneration – the #1 cause of blindness in people over 55 years – make sure to avoid taking aspirin. A major study linked aspirin to America's epidemic of macular degeneration. The so often prescribed one-aspirin-a day routine makes your retinas more likely to hemorrhage. Besides, aspirin belongs to the same class of painkillers as Vioxx, Celebrex and Aleve, all of which were found to increase heart attack and stroke risk by over 50%.]

Examinations have shown that by abstaining from food for a periodic length of time both fat cells and collagen fiber deposits begin to reduce in size and amount. This also demonstrates that overeating protein *does,* in fact, increase protein tissue in the body; the sites of the protein deposits being the basement membranes of the capillary walls and the connective tissues that surround the cells. As a direct consequence of this development, the thickened blood vessel walls are no longer capable of absorbing sufficient amounts of oxygen, water, and nutrients and removing all the metabolic waste products that the cells which constitute them produce. Hence, the cells that make up these blood vessels become injured and eventually die from malnutrition, suffocation, and dehydration.

In a young person, the blood vessels of the heart have a diameter of about 3mm. By regularly overeating protein foods, the normally smooth and polished inner wall of a blood vessel becomes uneven, and the blood vessel as a whole thickens and loses its elasticity. This leads to a deterioration of blood flow throughout the circulatory system, and may culminate in a complete blockage. Coronary arteries that are totally blocked resemble an old rusty, damaged, calcified water pipe. Their walls are brownish-red and are clogged up with yellowish, calcified material.

The Revealing Role of Homocysteine

Researchers discovered that the toxic, sulphur-containing amino acid *homocysteine* (HC) promotes the tiny clots that initiate arterial damage and the catastrophic ones that precipitate **most** heart attacks and strokes (Ann Clin & Lab Sci, 1991 and Lancet 1981). HC results from normal metabolism of the amino acid *methionine* – which is abundant in red meat (especially well done steak), milk, and dairy products. Normally, your body has a built-in defense mechanism against homocysteine buildup – it transforms it into a harmless substance called *cystathionine*, which is flushed from the body in the urine. However, regularly overeating proteins greatly undermines this ability.

Although the role of increased homocysteine levels in the blood as a major risk factor of heart disease has been common knowledge in the field of medical research for many years, it is only now being recognized as such in the field of applied medicine. The presence of unsafe levels of homocysteine in the body is thought to be associated with people who are genetically unable to convert homocysteine at a sufficient rate. But the enormous incidence of abnormal homocysteine levels among heart disease patients suggests that the genetic factor is secondary, or may even be a response to continuously overwhelming the body with protein foods[5]. Foods that are high in folic acid[6] have been shown to drastically lower homocysteine levels and thereby reduce the risk of cardiovascular disease.

Conclusion: If you regularly consume large quantities of animal protein, including meat, pork, poultry, fish, eggs, milk, cheese, etc., your body's ability to break down and safely remove all the protein or homocysteine becomes increasingly impaired (if it is not already naturally inefficient by constitution). Since excessive protein consumption thickens the blood and increases its risk of clotting, the body is forced to store the protein and the by-products of protein metabolism in the connective tissues under the skin as well as in the connective tissue of the organs and the basement/basal membranes of the capillary network. When the storage capacity of these membranes is exhausted, no more protein can

---

[5] Similar to the phenomenon of genetic mutation in cancerous growths. See specific information in _Cancer Is Not A Disease – It's A Survival Mechanism,_ by the author.

[6] See Chapter 7 of _Timeless Secrets of Health & Rejuvenation._

be deposited in the capillaries. If over-consumption of animal protein continues, the body begins to store the excessive protein in the walls of the arteries (see illustration 1). At this stage, the main coronary arteries become thickened, damaged, and inefficient. As they become occluded and cut off the oxygen supply to the heart, a heart attack occurs. Thus, the storage of excessive protein in the body acts like a "time bomb," ready to explode at any moment.

C-Reactive Protein Reveals the Truth

Continuous storage of excessive proteins in the blood vessel walls will eventually damage them. To help repair the damage and remove weak and injured cells, the body responds with inflammation. Inflammation is not a disease, but the body's basic emergency-response system. When the body is threatened by disease-causing germs, such as storage of proteins in the basal membranes of the blood vessel and subsequent buildup of protective fatty plaque in the arteries, the immune system dispatches large amounts of specialized cells to swarm and destroy the invader or potentially life-threatening obstructions. In the process of trying to fix the problem through inflammation, the immune cells cause multiple lesions that become increasingly unstable and may eventually rupture. When the body is unable to contain the bleeding resulting from a ruptured lesion, and any attempts to seal off the wound (s) fails, a heart attack or stroke occurs.

In a groundbreaking study published in the New England Journal of Medicine in 2002, doctors from Boston's Brigham and Women's Hospital showed that a simple blood test, called C-Reactive Protein (CRP), was able to predict which patients are most likely to suffer a heart attack or stroke. CPR measures the presence and intensity of inflammation in the walls of the blood vessels. Inflammation in the blood vessel walls is a much more accurate indicator of imminent heart trouble than measuring the concentrations of the "good" cholesterol (HDL) and the "bad" cholesterol (LDL) in the blood. This finding is very significant because half of all heart attacks occur in people with normal cholesterol levels. It not only shows that inflammation plays a key role in heart disease, but also in a wide range of other disorders involving the circulatory system, including arthritis, diabetes and cancer.

CRP is a protein produced by the liver in reaction to the immune system's inflammatory response. A simple blood test is able to detect this protein. Its concentration in the blood can determine how inflamed the heart arteries may be.

In the above study, the research team tracked the levels of both CRP and LDL ("bad" cholesterol) in nearly 28,000 women for eight years. According to the results of the study, women with high levels of CRP were twice as likely to have heart disease as those with high LDL. It also showed that many women who later suffered heart attacks would have been given a clean bill of health on the basis of their low LDL. Just relying on testing a person's cholesterol levels may is not enough, and may, in fact endanger his life.

CRP cannot be considered the ultimate testing kid for heart disease either, because it can jump as much as 10-fold when a person is fighting a cold or the flu. Infection includes an inflammatory response, and, therefore, the C-reactive protein is most likely to show up in the blood. However, this important piece of research shows that cholesterol testing is not what we should be focusing on if we want to save the lives of people who are at risk of heart disease. This is further substantiated by the most recent research showing that elevated blood cholesterol level cannot even be considered to be a major risk factor for heart attack (see *Risk Indications of a Heart Attack* below). Instead, focusing on the very causes of the inflammatory response will help us eradicate the incidence of heart disease, as well as arthritis and cancer.

How Heart Attacks Really Occur

Just cutting off oxygen supply to the heart may not be enough to destroy the heart. The heart is one of the most innovative and resilient organs in the body, and it requires a lot of abuse for it to die. When the basement or basal membranes of the capillaries and arteries can no longer guarantee sufficient supply of oxygen, sugar, and insulin to the cells of the heart muscles, their ability to contract and pump blood is greatly reduced. Just to continue their work without enough oxygen, the heart cells begin to ferment glucose to produce energy, but this (anaerobic) process produces lactic acid, which acidifies the muscle tissues.

To continue maintaining its pumping action, the heart employs an additional emergency measure to gain energy, which is to mobilize and break down fats. Yet, without using oxygen in the process, these fats turn into harmful, cell-destructive acids. Proteins also begin to be used to provide energy; the by-products are once again harmful fatty acids. Since the thickening of the connective tissues as well the lymph and blood capillaries in the heart begins obstructing normal elimination of metabolic waste, the heart muscles become intensely saturated with harmful acidic material. This may cause intense pain in the heart.

If uric acid, a waste product resulting from the breaking down of old cells, is retained in the tissues, gout occurs. The congestion leads to severe dehydration in the muscle cells, which prompts a group of cells known as *mast cells* to secrete the hormone *histamine* – a major water-regulating hormone in the body). When *histamine* passes over the sensitive pain nerves in the tissues, strong muscle pain results. If this form of muscle rheumatism occurs in the heart, it is called *Angina pectoris*. Both the acid accumulation and lack of oxygen lead to the death of the heart cells.

Heart attacks can occur in a number of ways:

1. The connective tissues surrounding the heart cells may become so densely congested that the heart cells simply die a painless death of suffocation.
2. In the case of an angina attack, it is acidification and low oxygenation of the heart muscles that destroys the heart.

3.   The basal membranes of the capillaries and arteries are blocked and can no longer supply oxygen to the heart. The part of the heart where the attack occurs is also the part where the storage capacity for protein was first exceeded.

4.   A blood clot breaks loose from a congested and injured blood vessel, enters the heart and blocks its oxygen supply.

New Studies Question Value of Opening Arteries

The new and emerging understanding of how heart attacks occur raises the question how valuable or useful it is to open blocked arteries. For one thing, the increasingly popular aggressive treatments of opening arteries – bypass surgery, angioplasty[7] and stents[8] – do little or nothing to prevent the recurrence of an occlusion. Although bypass surgery was found to extend the lives of some patients with severe

---

[7] Opening of arteries by pushing plaque back with a tiny balloon and then, often, holding it there with a stent

[8] Stents consists of wire cages that hold plaque against an artery wall; they can alleviate crushing chest pain. They can also rescue someone in the midst of a heart attack by holding the closed artery open.

illness, it does nothing to prevent heart attacks. Overall, none of the currently used surgical procedures have been shown to significantly lower the mortality rate from heart disease.

One of the main reasons for the poor success rate of these treatments is that the vast majority of heart attacks do not originate with obstructions that narrow arteries. To tackle the heart disease epidemic spreading in most industrialized nations like North America, preventative strategies are the only ones that make sense. But since they cost near to nothing (including eating less protein, regular exercise, early bedtimes, balanced meals and regular meal times, drinking enough water, avoiding junk foods, giving up smoking, reducing alcohol consumption, etc.), prioritization of preventative approaches versus treatment after the fact is economically not lucrative enough for those in charge of health care.

The old model of understanding heart disease is rapidly falling apart, much to the surprise of heart experts. "There has been a culture in cardiology that the narrowings were the problem and that if you fix them the patient does better," said Dr. David Waters, a cardiologist at the University of California at San Francisco. This theory made so much sense to the surgeons, cardiologists and laypeople that for decades hardly anyone questioned it, except those few (including myself) who were more interested in discovering the true causes of heart disease. The newest scientific discoveries now finally exposed this theory's major flaws, with little room for discussion.

Until recently[9], researchers believed that coronary disease is akin to sludge building up in a pipe. Plaque accumulates slowly, over decades, and once a coronary artery is blocked, no blood can get through to the heart and the patient suffers a heart attack. In order to prevent this catastrophe from happening, the most apparent rational "solution" to this problem was to perform bypass surgery or angioplasty to replace or open up the narrowed artery before it closed completely. The assumption that this would avert heart attacks and prolong life seemed indisputable. However, as medical research shows, this theory is no longer valid, and therefore, misleading. A study published in the New England Journal of Medicine by Coronary Artery Bypass Surgery Cooperative Study Group clearly demonstrated that the three-year survival rate for bypass surgery is the same as if no surgery was undertaken.

---

[9] This is not quite true, since as long ago as 1986, Dr. Greg Brown of the University of Washington at Seattle published a paper showing that heart attacks originated in areas of coronary arteries where there was too little plaque to be stented or bypassed.

According to numerous heart disease studies, most heart attacks do not occur because an artery is narrowed by plaque. Instead, researchers say, heart attacks occur when an area of plaque bursts, causing formation of a blood clot over the area and abruptly blocking blood flow. In fact, in 75 to 80 percent of cases, the plaque that breaks off was not obstructing an artery at all and would, therefore, not even be considered for bypass surgery or stenting. The dangerous type of plaque is soft and fragile, produces no symptoms and would not be seen as an obstruction to blood flow. For that reason, bypassing the hardened parts of an artery does nothing to lower the risk of a future heart attack. Is it surprising then that so many heart attacks are unexpected? Accordingly, a person may have no problem jogging one day, but suffer a heart attack (or stroke) the next. If a narrowed artery were the culprit, the person would not even be able to exercise due to severe chest pain.

Most heart patients have hundreds of vulnerable plaques in their arteries. Since it is impossible to replace all these injured, plaque-ridden sections, the current interventional procedures are pretty helpless to prevent heart attacks. Regardless, this doesn't mean there are less bypasses or stent operations performed. The multi-billion dollar stent-business has, in fact, become unstoppable.

Heart researchers and some cardiologists are becoming increasingly frustrated with the fact that their findings are not being taken seriously enough by the health practitioners and their patients. "There is just this embedded belief that fixing an artery is a good thing," said Dr. Eric Topol, an interventional cardiologist at the Cleveland Clinic in Ohio. It has almost become fashionable to have one's arteries fixed, just in case. Dr. Topol points out that more and more people with no symptoms are now getting stents. In 2004, over one million Americans opted for a stent operation.

Although many doctors know that the old theory no longer holds true, they feel pressured to opening blocked arteries anyway, regardless whether patients have symptoms or not. Dr. David Hillis, an interventional cardiologist at the University of Texas Southwestern Medical Center in Dallas, explained: "If you're an invasive cardiologist and Joe Smith, the local internist, is sending you patients, and if you tell them they don't need the procedure, pretty soon Joe Smith doesn't send patients anymore. Sometimes you can talk yourself into doing it even though in your heart of hearts you don't think it's right."

According to Dr. Topol, a patient typically goes to a cardiologist with a vague complaint like indigestion or shortness of breath, or because a scan of the heart indicated calcium deposits – a sign of atherosclerosis, or buildup of plaque. Doing his job, the cardiologist follows the standard procedures and puts the patient in the cardiac catheterization room, examining the arteries with an angiogram. If you live in a developed country like America and are middle-aged or older, you are most likely to have atherosclerosis, and the angiogram will show a narrowing. It will not take much convincing to tell you that you need a stent. "It's this train where you can't get off at any station along the way," Dr. Topol said. "Once you get on the train, you're getting the stents. Once you get in the cath lab, it's pretty likely that something will get done."

Dr. Hillis believes that it is ingrained in the American psyche that the value of medical care is directly related to how aggressive it is. Hillis has tried to explain the evidence to his patients, but with little success. "You end up reaching a level of frustration," he said. "I think they have talked to someone along the line who convinced them that this procedure will save their life. They are told if you don't have it done you are, quote, a walking time bomb."

Even more disquieting, Dr. Topol said, is that stenting can actually cause minor heart attacks in about 4 percent of patients. This means that out of the one-million stent patients in 2004, 40,000 ended up suffering heart damage from a procedure meant to prevent it, heart damage that they may never have developed without undergoing the procedure.

According to a new report (October 15, 2004) in the *New England Journal of Medicine*, the two stents that are currently approved by the Food and Drug Administration (FDA), the Cordis Cypher sirolimus-eluting stent and the Boston Scientific Taxus Express paclitaxel-eluting stent, have been associated with highly publicized adverse events after they were approved for marketing.

Bypass, angioplasty and stent operations are not about preventing heart attacks per se. The obvious purpose of the procedures is symptom relief. Patients are satisfied that "something" was done, relieved of the anxiety of dying from a sudden heart attack. In addition, the doctors are satisfied that their patients are happy. Of course, the drug industry is satisfied because the patients are doomed to taking expensive drugs for the rest of their lives.

Risk Indications of a Heart Attack

Most food-related blood vessel diseases, including heart attacks, stroke, rheumatism, and angina pectoris, are not primarily disorders of sugar and fat metabolism, but diseases resulting from protein storage. Eating too much protein food can be considered one of the greatest risk factors for developing any kind of disease. The thickening of the basal membranes of blood vessels and connective tissues caused by the storage of protein affects the very lives of all cells in the body. When and wherever in the body such congestion occurs, premature aging of cells and organs result. On the other hand, wherever the capillary walls maintain their porous, flexible nature and original thinness, cell nourishment and organ vitality continue throughout life.

Fat and *cholesterol* are not the primary blocking agents of blood vessel walls and, can therefore, not be considered to be the main cause of heart disease or any other disease in the body. Storage of protein in the blood vessel walls, on the other hand, is the common factor in all patients who suffer from alimentary (food-caused) atherosclerosis. Since most people in the advanced nations have consistently been consuming excessively large quantities of protein, particularly since World War II, coronary heart disease has become the leading cause of death in the developed world. As you will be able to see below, most of the leading risk elements of suffering a heart attack are directly or indirectly linked with high protein consumption and protein deposits in the blood vessel walls. The following are the indications of such risks:

1. *Thickening of blood as measured by Hemocrit (packed cell volume)*

The *Hemocrit* is the volume of red blood cells in one liter of whole blood, determined by a simple and cheap blood test. If it is above 42%, the risk of a heart attack increases. A healthy person has a Hemocrit of 35% to 40%. Under the assumption that the presence of larger quantities of protein in the blood is harmless, many doctors consider a volume of 44-50% to be still in the normal range; research, however, has shown that heart attacks were twice as high when the Hemocrit reached 49% compared to when it was 42%. The fact is that the higher the Hemocrit rises the greater is the risk of suffering a heart attack.

The question arises, why would the volume of red blood increase to beyond 40%? When the basal membranes and the intercellular tissues become thickened due to storage of excessive protein, blood flow slows down and becomes obstructed. This "naturally" increases the concentration of all blood values, including proteins, fats, and sugar. The thickening of the blood poses a great risk that affects all parts of the body. To deal with the dangerously high concentration of protein in the blood, the pancreas secretes extra insulin, but in doing so, the insulin may further injure and weaken the blood vessel walls. The cells making up the capillary walls start to absorb some the excessive protein, convert it into collagen, and deposit it in their basal membranes. Although this has a much-needed thinning effect on the blood, it also reduces nutrient transport to the cells. When the cells signal malnutrition, the blood nutrient levels begin to rise until the pressure of diffusion is high enough again to deliver enough nutrients to the cells.

In the meanwhile, this constant maneuvering raises the number of red blood cells, which contain the red colored *hemoglobin.* Hemoglobin combines with oxygen in the lungs and transports it to all the body cells. With increased thickness of the basal membranes, the oxygen supply to the cells also becomes restricted. The resulting increased need for oxygen by the cells raises hemoglobin concentrations in the red blood cells. However, this makes the red blood cells swell up. Eventually, they are too enlarged to pass through the tiny capillaries, blocking them altogether.

This even more drastically cuts down the nutrient and water supply to the cells, which subsequently begin to suffer dehydration. To signal dehydration, the cells release their water deficiency enzyme *renin* into the tissue fluid, which through a myriad of chemical events leads to an increase of heartbeat and cardiac output. This emergency measure increases water supply to the cells and prevents their demise, but it also raises the blood pressure. Known as *essential hypertension,* this situation causes even more stress and damage to the blood vessels than have already occurred. The vicious cycle is closed. The preconditions of suffering a heart attack are now in place.

Conclusion: Both factors combined – an increased Hemocrit, which indicates increased blood thickening, and a higher hemoglobin concentration in the red blood cells – reduce blood circulation. A round, red-colored face and chest are typical indications of an abnormally high blood volume and a decreased blood circulation in the adult hypertensive and diabetic patient. The cell tissues begin to dehydrate as water distribution becomes increasingly difficult. The rate and force of contraction of the heart muscle increases to help maintain the cardiac output against a sustained rise in congestion throughout the circulatory system. Eventually, the heart can no longer afford such strenuous activity and collapses.

2. *Eating too much Animal Protein*

The majority of heart attack patients confirm that they have been eating large quantities of animal protein, including, meat, chicken, fish, eggs, or cheese throughout their life or at least for many years. By contrast, there are virtually no heart attacks among vegetarians eating a balanced plant food diet.

3. *Cigarette Smoking*

The risk of cardiovascular diseases increases greatly with smoking. This, however, is not so much due to the nerve toxin *nicotine*, which is completely broken down within a few hours after smoking, but is rather caused by the *carbon oxide* (CO) contained in cigarette smoke. *Carbon oxide* or *monoxide* diffuses from the lungs into the blood where it attaches itself to the hemoglobin of the red cells, about 300 times faster and tighter than oxygen does. All the CO of the inhaled smoke combines with hemoglobin and thereby blocks off oxygen transport to the cells. The red blood cells, which are loaded with carbon monoxide-hemoglobin, begin to burst and shed their defective protein particles into the plasma of the blood from where many of them are deposited in the basal membranes of the capillary walls. When the capillaries' storage capacity has reached its saturation point, the arteries begin to deposit the protein debris in their walls.

This makes the carbon monoxide of cigarette smoke a slow-working, but lethal poison that, by forming excessive amounts of protein debris, destroys the body's circulatory network and heart muscles. In addition, passive smokers inhale large amounts of carbon monoxide, which explains why they are at a similar risk of developing coronary heart disease.

4. *Constitutional (genetic) Disposition towards Reduced Protein Breakdown*

People whose constitution does not require extra food protein in order to be healthy (mostly the *Kapha* and *Pitta* types)[10] do not have a very efficient enzyme system for breaking down food protein. Since constitutional body-types are mostly hereditary, this genetically determined "inefficiency" is passed on from parents to children. Those with a family history of heart attacks appear to be at risk because of possible hereditary factors, but the role of genetics in heart disease is only marginal. The primary reason is family members sharing a similar diet, lifestyle and

---

[10] To determine what body type you are, see author's book, *Timeless Secrets of Health & Rejuvenation.*

constitutional body type, with possibly the same "inefficient" enzyme systems for destroying excessive, unused proteins.

5. *Women during and after Menopause*

Women who consume large quantities of protein foods and/or smoke cigarettes are at risk once their menstrual cycles become irregular or come to an end. The regular loss of menstrual blood practically protects a woman (before menopause) from accumulating dangerous amounts of protein in the body, as long as the reproductive system functions normally. This may explain why menstruating women before age 40 are generally not at risk of suffering a heart attack, whereas men of that age are. All the different blood values in women under 40 are lower than among men in the same age group. These include red blood cells, hemoglobin, Hemocrit, and the total amount of protein. Research has shown that men aged between 30 and 40 years are six times more likely to die from a heart attack than women of the same age. In fact, heart attacks among menstruating women are extremely rare.

Once a woman's menstrual cycles subside, if she continues eating animal protein, the level of protein concentration in the blood begins to rise steadily. By the time she is about 50 years old, her risk of suffering a heart attack is nearly the same as it is for a man of the same age. The earlier the menopause begins the greater the risk. Women, whose ovaries have been removed before age 35, have a seven times greater risk of a heart attack than those who have yet to enter menopause.

The hot flushes and reddening of the face, which many women experience during menopause, are most often signs of higher blood values. They indicate that the body has stored excessive amounts of protein, which it can no longer expel with the menstrual blood. It has now been found that a diet consisting of a lot of dairy products hastens the forming of atherosclerotic deposits in a woman's body even further, and, as I will explain later, causes osteoporosis.

6. _Not eating enough fruit and vegetables; smoking; lack of exercise_

It was a wake-up call for Baby Boomers when newscasters were reporting in 2004 about emergency heart surgery performed on former President Bill Clinton. Unfortunately, the message conveyed to the world wasn't on improving heart health, but on taking the right drugs. It was by mere coincidence that just one week before President Clinton was admitted to the hospital, the prestigious medical journal *The Lancet* sounded a wakeup call with a different meaning. A major new study on heart disease risk published by the *Lancet* had this message for those concerned about their hearts: "Wake up and get heart healthy. You don't need medicine for that."

When President Clinton left office in 2001, he was still on the cholesterol-lowering statin drug *Zocor*. However, once his excessive weight came off and his cholesterol levels dropped, he discontinued taking the statin drug. When mainstream doctors heard about Clinton's heart condition, they immediately pointed the finger at not taking the statins as being the culprit. "See what happens when you don't take your pills?" Their words carried a warning for the rest of us who perhaps are just as careless when it comes to keeping our cholesterol levels in check. Some cardiologists believe that Clinton will now have to be on a much higher dose of a cholesterol-lowering drug for the rest of his life. This is certainly not unusual after undergoing a heart bypass operation, but it does not always make sense, and perhaps it hardly ever does.

In a *Newsday* report, Dr. Valavanur Subramanian, chairman of cardiovascular surgery at New York's Lenox Hill Hospital, noted that two of the three arteries used in Clinton's operation were mammary arteries, taken from his chest. Dr. Subramanian described these arteries as "extraordinarily resistant to cholesterol buildup." The question arises why put a man on potentially dangerous statin drugs when his arteries are virtually incapable of accumulating cholesterol deposits. Clinton is also most likely sentenced for life to taking a daily aspirin, along with a diuretic drug (to prevent buildup of fluid), and a beta blocker (to help regulate heartbeat). This potentially hazardous drug cocktail is going to be his "crutch" for the rest of his life, unnecessarily, though. According to the editors of the Lancet, the new study titled INTERHEART is one of the most robust studies ever done on heart disease risk factors. The 260 researchers closely observed and rigorously tested 15,000 heart attack patients for about a decade, matching them with the same number of subjects who had not experienced any heart problems. The worldwide study included male and female subjects with a wide range of ages, cultural backgrounds and dietary habits. The result may come as a shock to those who believe that high LDL cholesterol (the "bad" cholesterol), is a major risk factor for heart attacks. According to the study this isn't the case.

According to INTERHEART, the number one physical risk factor of heart attack is an abnormal ratio of *apolipoproteinB (apoB)* to *(apoA1)*. Apolipoprotein is cholesterol's protein component. ApoB is the protein found in LDL, and apoA1 is found in HDL. The ideal apo ratio is one apoB to two apoA1. In other words, an elevated bad cholesterol (LDL) alone poses no major risk for the heart. Yet, high LDL is the very condition cholesterol-lowering statin drugs are prescribed for. The whole focus has been on getting your cholesterol down and keeping it low. When doing this with drugs, you are asking for trouble. Thus, due to the numerous harmful side-effects of statin drugs, millions of unsuspecting healthy people have already been turned into real patients with real (drug-caused) diseases. They have never been told that elevated cholesterol poses no major risk to their heart. Certainly, no patient I know has heard from his doctor about the apo ratio.

The INTERHEART study was launched in 1994, at a time other major risk factors were not yet widely known; factors such as triglycerides, homocysteine and C-reactive protein. In their report the INTERHEART team listed the most important risks of heart attack

44

after apo ratio (from greater to lesser risk): cigarette smoking, diabetes, high blood pressure, excessive abdominal fat, stress, inadequate intake of fruits and vegetables, and lack of exercise. Much to the surprise of the cholesterol/heart disease lobbyists, elevated cholesterol wasn't one of them. In the concluding remarks of the 10-year study, researchers wrote that the relative risk for heart attack can be lowered by about 80 percent just by doing three things: eating plenty of fruits and vegetables, getting regular exercise, and avoiding smoking. Since cholesterol-lowering drugs have not been shown to lower the risk of heart attack, they were notably absent in the study's list of recommendations, much to the annoyance of the major statin producers.

INTERHEART is not the only large study that discovered the significance of the apo ratio. During a Swedish study, researchers tracked more than 175,000 men and women for about five and a half years. The average age of the subjects was 48. Researchers studied all the main markers believed to be a risk, including total cholesterol, LDL and HDL cholesterol, triglycerides, and concentrations of apoB and apoA1. Over the course of the study, 864 men and 359 women died from heart attacks. While comparing the blood profiles of these heart attack victims to the remainder of the participants, the researchers found that an unbalanced apo ratio was the strongest predictor of heart attack death among all of the markers studied. Apo ratio was the only marker consistent over all age groups. They also found that an abnormal apo ratio continued to pose the same heart attack risk even when total cholesterol, LDL cholesterol, and triglycerides were within normal ranges.

It is my experience with hundreds of heart disease patients that eliminating animal proteins from their diet has helped restore normal heart functions, sometimes within a matter of six weeks. I, therefore, have come to the conclusion that eating a high protein diet, which is among the most acid-forming diets anyone can eat, greatly upsets the apo ratio and induces an inflammatory response in the coronary arteries. Both factors go hand in hand and, as we now know, pose the greatest physical risks to the health of the heart.

7. *Kidney Disease*

Just as is the case with congestion of the liver's bile ducts and gallbladder with stones, many people live with undetected, chronic kidney disease. When symptoms finally begin to appear, it is often too late to reverse the damage. Health officials estimate that there are many as 10 to 20 million people in the U.S.

with serious kidney problems. However, you may ask what this has to do with heart disease.

Two new studies, published in September 2004 in the New England Journal of Medicine (NEJM), found a clear correlation between chronic kidney disease (even non-severe) and cardiovascular disease, which makes prevention of kidney disease more important than ever.

In one of the studies, researchers examined three years of data covering the medical records from over one million patients (made available to them by the Kaiser Permanente Renal Registry in San Francisco). The average age of the subjects was 52 years. The research team specifically looked at the results of a blood test that measures the rate at which kidneys are able to filter waste from the bloodstream (glomerular filtration rate or GFR). The findings revealed that as GFR dropped, the risks of cardiovascular disease, stroke, hospitalization and death all increased sharply. In those patients where the GFR was below 45, the risk of death jumped by 17 percent, and the risk of a cardiovascular event increased by more than 40 percent.

In the second study, conducted in the cardiovascular division of Boston's Brigham and Women's Hospital, researchers showed that a GFR below 45 among patients who had suffered heart attack boosted death risk to more than 45 percent. Noting that factors common to kidney disease (such as the protein albumin in the urine, high homocysteine levels, inflammation and anemia) may boost the risk of cardiovascular disease and death, the researchers concluded that even mild kidney disease should be considered a major risk factor for cardiovascular complications after a heart attack.

To ensure that your kidneys continue functioning properly, you will need to keep your colon, liver and kidneys clean[11]. Kidney health largely depends on efficient performance of the digestive system. In addition, to allow the kidneys do their important job of blood filtering, the basal membranes of the capillaries and arteries supplying blood to the kidney cells must be free of any protein deposits. Kidney health also depends on how well the lymph ducts are able to drain the kidneys' metabolic waste products and millions of turned-over, dead kidneys cells each day. Congestion in the body's largest lymph vessel (thoracic duct) leads to back-flushing of waste in the kidneys, which slowly suffocates them in their own waste and cell debris. Among the most lymph-congesting foods are animal proteins, milk and

---

[11] See *The Amazing Liver & Gallbladder Flush* by the author.

cheese, as well as highly processed and fat-deprived foods.

Besides keeping the main eliminative organs clean, there are other ways to prevent kidney disease, including: a nutritious low-protein diet, regular nutritious meals, sleeping between 10 p.m. – 6 a.m. to permit the liver and kidneys to do their respective work, taking care of one's emotional health, and most other advice provided in this book. If you keep your kidneys healthy, your heart may have little to fear.

8. *Antibiotics and other synthetic drugs*

It is becoming increasingly evident that medicinal drugs that have a suppressive effect on anything in the body diminish heart health. Every time you try to prevent the body from clearing out accumulated toxins and waste through a cold, a viral infection, or a disease process that includes inflammation, your heart is burdened with the difficult task of having to push the harmful waste material released from the tissues back to where it came from. With each new attempt to subdue pain, infection, cholesterol, etc., less and less of this waste finds its way out of the body. Some of it ends up congesting the lymph ducts responsible for draining the heart muscles of their metabolic waste products. Antibiotics are one of the leading culprits for this form of heart damage.

For many years, antibiotics have been over-prescribed, often for infections (such as the common cold and flu) that they have no effect on at all. It is common knowledge that antibiotics don't kill viruses, only bacteria. Now a new study shows that the popular antibiotic *erythromycin,* which has been widely used since the 1950s, may actually trigger cardiac arrest.

For many years, heart doctors have been aware of a risk of cardiac arrest when erythromycin is used intravenously, but this risk has been less well known among family practitioners who often prescribe the same antibiotic in pill form to treat a wide variety of infections. This new study, conducted by researchers from Vanderbilt University, examined the risk of cardiac arrest when oral erythromycin is used alone or with other medications. Their report, which was published in the New England Journal of Medicine in October 2004, covered the medical records of more than 4,400 Medicaid patients, averaging 15 years per patient. About 1,475 subjects suffered cardiac arrest during the study period. When the complete medication use of each subject was analyzed, researchers came up with these results:

- The rate of sudden death from cardiac causes was twice as high among patients using erythromycin, compared to subjects that didn't use the antibiotic.
- Two blood pressure medications that are sold generically – verapamil and diltiazem – were both associated with an additional increased risk of cardiac arrest when taken with erythromycin.
- Other drugs associated with increased cardiac attack risk when taken with erythromycin include the antibiotic clarithromycin, the vaginal yeast infection drug fluconazole, and two antifungal drugs: itraconazole and ketoconazole

According to the researchers, blood levels of these additional drugs may be boosted by erythromycin, making the blood thick and sluggish. This can result in a slower heart rate, which in turn may trigger irregular rhythms, setting in motion a cardiac arrest. In an interview with The Associated Press, the lead researcher of the study, Wayne A. Ray, Ph.D., warned that erythromycin levels may also be increased by drinking grapefruit juice or by taking protease inhibitors used to treat AIDS.

Just because your doctor prescribes you a medical drug does not mean it is safe. Very few drug interactions with other drugs or with common foods have ever been tested. Drug prescription can be a gamble of life and death that you a willing to risk when you enter your doctor's office. The bottom line is that all pharmaceutical drugs contain poisons that have a detrimental effect on your health. Your heart is the one that pays the ultimate price for the constantly offered and highly praised shortcuts to health.

The fact is no Disease Control Agency or Federal Drug Administration (FDA) can protect you from developing a serious illness or dying as a result of using prescribed drugs. The VIOXX scandal of September 2004 has taught us that there are no safe drugs out there. VIOXX, a leading arthritis drug, was withdrawn by its producer, Merck & Co, after evidence leaked out that its use doubled the risk of heart attack and stroke. [As per the end of 2004, Merck was faced with over 1,000 lawsuits]. According to documentation, this risk has been known to both the drug producer and the FDA since the mid-nineties. The result of this well-kept secret was that a minimum of 27,000 people suffered a heart attack or died because of it. Given the high number of unreported side-effects, this number may well exceed hundreds of thousands.

More are more drugs are coming under suspicion of being killer drugs. Bextra is next.

According to a study of more than 1,500 patients who had previously undergone cardiac surgery, those who were treated for pain with Bextra were more likely to have heart and blood clotting problems than those who received no drug at all. Stroke, heart attack, blood clots in the lung, deep vein blood clots in the leg, all can result just from taking this drug. Arthritis drugs have never been safe, but they have never been properly tested for safety. Vioxx, Celebrex, Bextra, Aleeve, Aspirin are just plain poisons. Another arthritis drug – *infliximab* (Remicade) – is on cancer-causing alert. Amazingly, so many people have been so blinded by clever advertising campaigns and methods of brainwashing that they have no clue they are methodically poisoned in order to support and sustain, besides oil, the most lucrative business in the world – the pharma-medical industry.

The main question is how could anyone possibly want to entrust his life to the hands of drug-producers whose only objective it is to keep the sickness-business going by making sure what they produce creates more health problems that it can resolve? In the majority of all cases, attempting to prescribe medications that claim to offer a relief to the symptoms of disease is not only a dangerous approach, but also an unscientific and unethical one.

Ending the Cholesterol -Heart Disease Myth

At no time has there been a record of cholesterol ever having blocked a vein in the body! It is not the stickiness of cholesterol that causes the blockage of healthy blood vessel walls! The body uses cholesterol as a kind of bandage to cover abrasions and tears in its arterial walls. It is a life-saver.

For the past thirty-five years, the lipoprotein *cholesterol* has been stigmatized to be the number one cause for most deaths in the rich nations – heart disease. This is how the theory goes: cholesterol is known to increase in the blood stream of many people today, stick to the walls of arteries, and eventually starve the heart muscles of oxygen and nutrients. The masses are advised to reduce or ban fats like butter and oils from their diet so that they can live without the fear of dying from a heart attack. The tremendous concern of being attacked by this "vicious" lipoprotein has finally led to innovative technologies that can even extract cholesterol from cheese, eggs, and sausages, thus making these "deadly" foods "consumer-safe." Products that claim to be low in cholesterol, such as margarine and light-foods, have become a popular choice of "healthy eating."

54

Cholesterol –
Not the Culprit After All

As INTERHEART and other studies have shown, cholesterol isn't even a major risk factor for heart disease. An earlier study sponsored by the German Ministry of Research and Technology showed that there is no exact link between food cholesterol and blood cholesterol. Even more surprising, in Japan, the cholesterol levels have risen during recent years, yet the number of heart attacks has dropped. The largest health study ever conducted on the risks of heart disease took place in China. Like so many other similar studies, it found no connection between heart disease and the consumption of animal fats.

All the major European long-term cholesterol studies confirmed that a low fat diet did not reduce cholesterol levels by more than 4% percent, in most cases by merely 1-2%. Since measurement mistakes are usually higher than 4% and cholesterol levels naturally increase by 20% in autumn and drop again in winter, the anti-cholesterol campaigns since the late 1980s have been very misleading, to say the least. A more recent study from Denmark involving 20,000 men and women, in fact, demonstrated that most heart patients have normal cholesterol levels. The bottom line is that cholesterol hasn't been proved a risk factor for anything.

The current medical understanding of the cholesterol issue is more than incomplete. The argument that animal tests on rabbits have confirmed that fatty foods cause hardening of the arteries sounds reasonable, but only when the following facts are omitted:

1. Rabbits respond 3,000 times more sensitively to cholesterol than humans do.
2. Rabbits, which are non-carnivorous animals by nature, are force-fed excessive quantities of egg yolk and brain for the sake of proving that cholesterol-containing foods are harmful.
3. The DNA and enzyme systems of rabbits are not designed for consumption of fatty foods, and if given a choice, these animals would never eat eggs or brains.

Death in Trans Fatty Acids

It is obvious that the arteries of these animals have only an extremely limited ability to respond to the damage caused by such unsuitable diets. For over three and half decades the Western civilization assumed that animal fats are the main cause of dietary heart disease. This misinformation is highlighted by the fact that heart attacks began to rise when consumption of animal fats actually decreased. This was verified by British research, which revealed that those areas in the UK where people consumed more margarine and less butter had the highest numbers of heart attacks. Further studies revealed that heart attack patients had consumed the least amounts of animal fats.

In this context, it is important to differentiate between processed and unprocessed fats. It has been discovered that people who died from a heart attack were found to have many more of the harmful fatty acids, which are derived from the partially hydrogenated vegetable oils of margarine, in their fat tissue than those who survived. These so-called "faulty" fats (trans-fatty acids) envelop and congest the cellular membranes, including those of the heart and the heart arteries. This practically starves the cells of oxygen, nutrients, and water, and eventually kills them. In another more comprehensive study, 85,000 nurses working in American hospitals observed a higher risk for heart disease in patients who consumed margarine, crisps, biscuits, cakes, and white bread, all of which contain "faulty" fatty acids.

Eating margarine can increase heart disease in women by 53% over eating the same amount of butter according to a recent Harvard Medical Study. While increasing LDL cholesterol, margarine lowers the beneficial HDL cholesterol. It also increases the risk of cancers by up to five fold. Margarine suppresses both the immune response and insulin response. This highly processed and artificial product is but one molecule from being plastic. Flies, bacteria, fungi, etc. won't go near it because it has no nutritional value and cannot be broken down by them. It can last for years, not just outside the body, but inside as well. It is very apparent that eating damaged, rancid fats or trans-fats can destroy any healthy organism and should be avoided.

As early as 1956, The Lancet cautiously warned that *"...coronary artery disease becomes in part a preventable disorder, but at the cost of a complete revolution in our present-day dietary habits. The hydrogenation plants of our modern food industry may turn out to have contributed to the causation of a major disease.* "The persistent ignoring of this fact by governments and doctors can be held responsible for the unnecessary death of millions of people in the past five decades.

Let's summarize the most important points made above:

- It is very damaging advice to "keep your fats low." To digest fats properly and make good use of them we need 15

– 20% of our food to be in fat, natural fats and oils.

- If you want to get rid of excessive fat in your body, you need to eat more of those natural fats and avoid the unhealthy, toxic fats. Not eating natural fats slows your digestion and metabolism and, therefore, actually makes you accumulate fat. Farm animals that are deprived of fats and fed with carbohydrates become hungrier, eat more and put on fat more quickly. Every cell in our body needs healthy fat derived from the essential fatty acids.

- The body has no capacity to process and utilize margarine and hydrogenated oils. Eating these unnatural fats will clog up cell membranes, arteries, the heart, cause cancer and impair brain development in children and in adults. Researchers consider them a leading cause of death. Hence, sales are controlled or forbidden in Europe. The English speaking countries, though, have resisted the ban on these Frankenstein foods due to the enormous pressure by the manufacturing industry.

Healthy Today – Sick Tomorrow

Unfortunately, elevated cholesterol, also referred to as *hypercholesterolemia,* has become the dominating health risk of the 21st century. It is actually an invented disease that doesn't show up as one. Even the healthiest people may have elevated serum cholesterol and yet they remain healthy. Nevertheless, they are instantly turned into patients when a routine blood test reveals that they have a "cholesterol problem."

Since feeling good is actually a symptom of high cholesterol, the cholesterol issue has confused millions of people. To be declared sick when you actually feel great is a hard nut to swallow. Therefore, it may take a lot of effort on a behalf of a practicing physician to convince his patients that they are sick and need to take one or more expensive drugs for the rest of their lives. It may actually have a depressing effect on these healthy individuals to be told that apart from having to take side effect causing drugs to lower their cholesterol levels, they also learn that they will require regular checkups and blood tests. The worry-free, good life is now over.

These doctors cannot be blamed for the blunder of converting healthy people into patients. Behind them stands the full force of the U.S. government, the media and the medical establishment, agencies, and pharmaceutical companies, to name a few. Each has contributed to create relentless pressure to disseminate the cholesterol dogma and convince the population that high cholesterol is its number one enemy. We are told that we need to combat it, by all means, to keep us safe from the dreadful consequences of hypercholesterolemia.

What constitutes a healthy level of cholesterol has been revised repeatedly during the past 25 years, which certainly does not give me much confidence in a system of medicine that professes to be founded on scientific principles. In the early days of measuring cholesterol levels, a person at risk was any middle-aged man whose cholesterol is over 240 with other risk factors, such as smoking or being overweight.

After the adjustment of parameters during the Cholesterol Consensus Conference in 1984, the population was hit by a shock wave. Now, anyone (male or female) with overall cholesterol readings of 200 mg% (200mg per 100 ml) could receive the dreaded diagnosis and a prescription for pills. The claim that 200 blood *serum cholesterol* is normal and everything above is dangerous scientifically unfounded, though. At least, this is what all the major cholesterol studies showed. In fact, in a 1995 issue of the Journal of the American Medical Association, it reported that there was no evidence linking high cholesterol levels in women with heart conditions later in life. Although it is considered completely normal for a 55-year-old woman to have a *cholesterol* level of 260 mg%, most women that age are not told about this. Healthy employees are found to have an average of 250 mg% with high fluctuations in both directions.

The lack of evidence linking elevated cholesterol with increased risk of heart disease, however, didn't stop the brainwashing of the masses. From one day to the next, 84% of all the men and 93% of all the women aged 50-59 in the U.S. whose *cholesterol* levels are 220 mg% and more, were suddenly told they needed treatment for heart disease. The completely unsubstantiated, but rigorously promoted cholesterol theories turned most of us into patients for a disease that we probably will never develop. Fortunately, not everyone has followed the advice to have their cholesterol levels checked.

To make matters worse, the official, acceptable cholesterol level has now been moved down to 180. If you already have had a heart attack once, your cardiologist will tell you to take cholesterol-lowering statins even if your cholesterol is very low. From the viewpoint of conventional medicine, having a heart attack implies that your cholesterol must be too high. Hence, you are being sentenced to a lifetime of statins and a boring low-fat diet. Even if you have not experienced any heart trouble yet, you are already being considered for possible treatment. Since so many children now show signs of elevated cholesterol, we have a whole new generation of candidates for medical treatment. So yes, current edicts stipulate cholesterol testing and treatment for young adults and even children. The statin drugs that doctors use to push cholesterol levels down are *LIPITOR* (atorvastatin), *Zocor* (simvastatin), *Mevacor* (lovastatin), and *Pravachol* (pravastatin). If you decide to follow your doctor's advice and take one of these drugs make certain to read the list of side-effects so that you know the risks you are taking.

If you want to obtain objective and untainted information on cholesterol, agencies like the National Institutes of Health and the American College of Cardiology are certainly not the places from which to obtain it. Until not too long ago, they wanted you to keep your overall level below 150. Then, in 2001, they finally admitted that measuring overall cholesterol levels makes no sense at all. Therefore, they began recommending keeping LDL levels below 100. Now their aim is to keep LDL lower than 70. Every time they lower the target, the number of "patients" requiring treatment jumps dramatically. Being officially backed by these agencies, doctors feel motivated, if not obliged, to prescribe these expensive drugs to these new patients. The extensive promotional campaigns by the pharmaceutical giants have already brainwashed the masses to believe they need these drugs to be safe from sudden heart attack. Even if a doctor knows the truth about the cholesterol issue, these anxious patients will demand a prescription from him. That the massive sales of these best-selling drugs of all time drive up health care costs to levels that undermine economic growth and make basic health care unaffordable to an ever-increasing number of people doesn't seem to be their immediate concern.

In 2004, there were already 36 million statin candidates in the U.S., with 16 million using LIPITOR alone. When the official LDL target level drops to 70, there will be another 5 million people eligible for their use. At the consumer markup price of $272.37 and a cost of $5.80 for a month supply of LIPITOR, for example, you can do the math and understand the incentive the pharmaceutical industry has to push their products and make them a mass commodity.

What Statins May do to You!

Statins inhibit the production of cholesterol. Now, most people would think that this is a good thing. The statins manage to lower cholesterol by inhibiting the body's production of *mevalonate*, which is a precursor of cholesterol. When the body makes less mevalonate, less cholesterol is produced by the cells and thus blood cholesterol goes down as well. This still sounds good to most people. However, mevalonate is a precursor of other substances, too, substances with many important biologic functions that you definitely don't want to disrupt (see side effects below).

The masses are told that the most important objective is to get rid of the excessive cholesterol so that it doesn't clog up their arteries and cause a heart attack. This simplistic train of thought caused the trouble in the first place. Contrary to what we know about the true value of cholesterol, it has been declared to us that this essential substance is a dangerous nuisance that makes our lives miserable.

The fact is that each cell in your body requires cholesterol to make it waterproof and prevent its membrane from becoming leaky or porous. If your diet, for example, contains a lot of acidic compounds, such as meat protein, sugar and trans fats, your cell membranes become damaged and require repair. To fulfill the repair request by the cells, the body releases a flood of corticoid hormones that cause extra amounts of cholesterol to be transported to areas where needed.

One of cholesterol's many roles is to repair tissue damage. Scar tissue is known to contain high levels of cholesterol, including scar tissue in the arteries. In other words, whenever an artery becomes injured due to acid attacks and buildup of proteins in their walls, you can expect cholesterol to be there to help repair the damage as best as possible. The increased demand for more cholesterol is naturally met by the liver, which can raise production by 400% if necessary. That this emergency response must lead to elevated cholesterol levels in the blood is not only common sense, but also desirable. Obviously, this changes any negative preconceived notions that you may have had about the role of cholesterol in your body. Cholesterol is not your worst enemy, but your best friend.

Apart from cholesterol protecting your health, there are many more reasons why we need to avoid meddling with the finely tuned cholesterol-producing mechanism in the body (explained in following sections). A real problem arises when we lower cholesterol by bypassing or disturbing this life-essential mechanism. The cholesterol-lowering statin drugs do just that. If your body has reasons to increase cholesterol levels in your blood, it is for your protection only. Artificially lowering blood cholesterol with synthetic drugs removes that protection and can generate an entire host of health problems, starting with disrupting the production of adrenal hormones. This, in turn, can lead to:

- Blood sugar problems
- Edema
- Mineral deficiencies
- Chronic inflammation
- Difficulty in healing
- Allergies
- Asthma
- Reduced libido
- Infertility
- Various reproductive disorders
- Brain damage

The last side-effect on the list – brain damage – may be one of the most disturbing side-effects resulting from long-term use of stains. A case-control study published in 2002 by the American Academy of Neurology found that long-term exposure to statins may substantially increase the risk of polyneuropathy.

The problem with statin drugs is that they *don't* cause immediate side-effects like the older, cholesterol-lowering drugs did. The old method used was to lower cholesterol by preventing its absorption from the gut, which led to nausea, indigestion, and constipation. Nevertheless, the old drugs' success rate was minimal and patient compliance was very low. Statin drugs became an overnight success story because they were able to lower cholesterol levels by 50 points or more, with no immediate major side-effects. On the false notion that cholesterol causes heart disease, statins – the bestselling pharmaceuticals of all time – have become the miracle drug of the 21st century. The promise of the drug giants is that if you keep taking their drugs for the rest of your life you will forever be protected against man's greatest killer disease. This equation, however, has two major flaws in it. One, cholesterol has never been proved to cause heart disease. Two, by lowering cholesterol with the help of statins, you can actually make your body very ill. The industry is now faced with an ever-growing number of reports listing the side effects that manifest many months after the commencement of therapy.

A 1999 study at St. Thomas' Hospital in London found that 36 percent of patients on LIPITOR's highest dose reported side effects and 10% of the patients at the lowest dose also reported side effects. The steady increase of obvious and hidden side-effects (such as liver damage) isn't at all surprising. The "benefits" (of lowering cholesterol) seen with LIPITOR early in the trial that led to its approval were so convincing that it was halted approximately two years ahead of schedule. The trial was never long enough to show that LIPITOR had long-term side-effects that could devastate people's lives. Side-effects from using LIPITOR include gas, stomach pain or cramps, diarrhea, constipation, heartburn, headache, blurred vision, dizziness, rash or itching, upset stomach, muscle pain, tenderness, muscle cramps or weakness with or without a fever.

The most commonly experienced side effects are muscle pain and weakness. Dr. Beatrice Golomb of San Diego, California is currently conducting a series of studies on statin side effects. Golomb found that 98 percent of patients taking LIPITOR and one-third of the patients taking Mevachor (a lower-dose statin) suffered from muscle problems, such as severe calf pain and foot pain. An increasing number of long-term patients (after three years) develop slurred speech, balance problems and severe fatigue. It often begins with restless sleep patterns. Fine motor skills can be affected and cognitive functions decline. Memory loss is not uncommon. Usually, when patients discontinue taking the statins, the symptoms weaken or disappear.

A new German study published in the July 25, 2005 issue of *The New England Journal of Medicine* found that not only do cholesterol-lowering statin drugs fail to help patients with severe diabetes, but statins may also double their risk of experiencing a deadly stroke.

I found in my own practice that regular statin users accumulate an excessive amount of cholesterol stones in the bile ducts of their liver and gallbladder, which can lead to a vast number of chronic diseases (see *The Amazing Liver & Gallbladder Flush* for details).

Before deciding to take LIPITOR (or other statins), there are some basic of points for you to consider:

- o You need to tell your doctor and pharmacist if you are allergic to LIPITOR/ Atorvastatin or any other drugs. *This obviously raises the question how many patients follow that advice.*
- o You are supposed to tell your doctor and pharmacist what prescription and nonprescription medications you are taking, especially antacids; antifungal medications such as itraconazole (Sporanox) and ketoconazole (Nizoral); digoxin (Lanoxin); erythromycin;

medications that suppress the immune system such as cyclosporine (Neoral, Sandimmune); oral contraceptives (birth control pills); other cholesterol-lowering medications such as cholestyramine (Questran), colestipol (Colestid), gemfibrozil (Lopid), and niacin (nicotinic acid); and vitamins. *You may wonder how many people follow that advice, and how many doctors ask this information of their patients?*

o You need to tell your doctor if you have or have ever had liver or kidney disease, a severe infection, low blood pressure, or seizures. *How many people actually know if their liver's bile ducts are packed with stones, whether their kidneys have major stone deposits in them, or if their blood pressure is below acceptable?*

o Tell your doctor if you are pregnant, plan to become pregnant, or are breast-feeding. If you become pregnant while taking LIPITOR/Atorvastatin, you are supposed to stop taking LIPITOR/atorvastatin and call your doctor immediately as this drug can harm the fetus. *If the drug can harm the fetus, you may need to ask what else it can harm.*

71

- o If you are having surgery, including dental surgery, tell the doctor or dentist that you are taking LIPITOR/Atorvastatin. *How many people remember to do that?*
- o Talk to your doctor about the safe use of alcohol while taking this LIPITOR drug. Alcohol increases the side effects caused by LIPITOR/Atorvastatin. *Many doctors forget to tell their patients about the potential risks regarding alcohol, and many patients just ignore that warning, often with severe consequences.*
- o Plan to avoid unnecessary or prolonged exposure to sunlight and to wear protective clothing, sunglasses, and sunscreen. LIPITOR/Atorvastatin may make your skin sensitive to sunlight. *It is a pretty serious condition when the sun becomes so dangerous that you have to hide from it.*
- o For the drugs to be effective, you also need to eat a low-cholesterol, low-fat diet. This kind of diet includes cottage cheese, fat-free milk, fish (not canned in oil), vegetables, poultry, egg whites, and polyunsaturated oils and margarines (corn, safflower, canola, and soybean oils). Avoid foods with excess fat in them such as meat (especially liver and

fatty meat), egg yolks, whole milk, cream, butter, shortening, lard, pastries, cakes, cookies, gravy, peanut butter, chocolate, olives, potato chips, coconut, cheese (other than cottage cheese), coconut oil, palm oil, and fried foods. *Please see Chapter 14 about the damaging side-effects that arise from being on a prolonged low-fat diet or light-food diet.*

But Doesn't Aspirin Protect Against Heart Disease?

If you are diagnosed with heart failure and follow the recommended treatment of taking blood thinners such as *aspirin* or *coumadin*, you could seriously endanger your health. In a recent study, researchers compared Blood-Thinning Therapies to no Antithrombotic Therapy. They not only found no advantage in undergoing such treatments, but risks of further complications. Participants included 279 patients who were diagnosed with heart failure that required diuretic therapy. The subjects were divided into three groups, aspirin therapy, warfarin therapy and no antithrombotic therapy.

Results of the Study

- Aspirin and warfarin didn't provide the patients with any valuable health benefits
- There didn't appear to be any substantial differences of incidences of death, nonfatal heart attacks or nonfatal stroke in the three groups of the study
- Patients in the aspirin group had increased chances of experiencing serious gastrointestinal problems
- Cases of minor bleeding complications were primarily seen among the aspirin and warfarin group
- Patients in the aspirin therapy group were twice as likely as the patients in the warfarin group to face hospitalization for cardiovascular complications, particularly worsening cases of heart failure during the first 12 months following the study
- Warfarin proved to be ineffective and should be eliminated as a treatment option

Based on the results from this study, the treatment of heart failure should not involve the use of drug-based blood thinners, such as aspirin. It is relatively easy to keep the blood thin through a balanced vegetarian diet, drinking sufficient quantities of water, avoiding diuretic foods and beverages, keeping regular meal and bedtimes, and cleansing the liver, kidneys and colon.

Dangers of Low Cholesterol

It seems we need to be more concerned about low cholesterol, which is a major risk for cancer, mental illness, stroke, suicide, liver diseases, anemia, and AIDS. Studies conducted in major German hospitals verified that low cholesterol levels are linked to high mortality rates. When cholesterol levels dropped to 150 mg%, two out of three patients died. Most of the patients whose cholesterol levels were high recovered from whatever they suffered. In addition, longevity in old homes is linked with higher levels of cholesterol. Recent studies published in the British Medical Journal (BMJ) indicate that a low level of blood cholesterol could increase a person's risk of suicide.

A study published in the Lancet in 1997 showed that particularly among the elderly, high total cholesterol levels are associated with longevity. The research suggests that elderly people with elevated cholesterol levels live longer and are less likely to die from cancer or infection. Doctors at Reykjavik Hospital and Heart Preventive Clinic in Iceland noted that the major epidemiological studies on cholesterol had not included the elderly. So when they studied total mortality and blood cholesterol in those over 80, they found that that men with blood cholesterol levels over 6.5 had less than half the mortality of those whose cholesterol level was around the 5.2 we are told is "healthy". In support of this discovery, scientists working at the Leiden University Medical Centre found that "each 1 mmol/l increase in total cholesterol corresponded to a 15% decrease in mortality." A study of Maori in New Zealand showed that those with the *lowest* levels of blood cholesterol had the *highest* mortality.

Similar findings were also borne out by the Framingham Heart Study. Forty years after the Framingham Heart Study began, its researchers looked at total mortality and cholesterol. They found *"no increased overall mortality with either high or low serum cholesterol levels"* among men over forty-seven years of age. There was also no relationship with women older than forty-seven or younger than forty. However, the researchers concluded that people whose cholesterol levels are falling may be at increased risk.

The same applies also to children. Research on seven to nine-year-old boys from six

76

countries revealed a strong correlation between low blood cholesterol and childhood deaths in those countries. The death rate rose dramatically as blood cholesterol levels fell. Therefore, for children too, low blood cholesterol is outright unhealthy. Once again, the official line is for parents to reduce their children's fat intake in order to lower their cholesterol or keep it low. Instead of telling the people to keep their cholesterol levels down, parents should be told that it is better to let cholesterol rise. This effectively lowers their risk of disease and death.

The low cholesterol-cancer connection has been known for many years. Moreover, although there never has been any convincing evidence that raised levels of cholesterol have any causal relationship with coronary heart disease, this hasn't stopped the drug giants from advertising statins drugs as a safe approach to protect the masses against heart disease. The extremist attempt to indiscriminately lower cholesterol levels, especially among the elderly where elevated cholesterol levels are normal and very necessary, has led to numerous cancers in the U.S. and worldwide. As most studies have shown, high serum cholesterol is a weak risk factor or no risk factor at all, for men above fifty, and actually increases longevity in those over eighty.

Women, in particular should be cautious about using statins. Most studies have shown that high serum cholesterol is not a risk factor for women at all, and, therefore, should not be lowered by any means. The bottom line is that cholesterol protects the body against cancer. Removing this natural protection is synonymous with "involuntary suicide." Both animal and human trials have demonstrated increases in cancers when cholesterol was lowered through fibrates and statins. In the CARE trial, for example, the relative breast cancer increase was a whooping 1,400%!

Then there is the low cholesterol-stroke connection. On Christmas Eve, 1997, a very important study made it to the headlines in the press. Researchers heading the famous Framingham study (still continuing) said that *"Serum cholesterol level is not related to incidence of stroke . . ."* and showed that for every three percent more energy from fat eaten, strokes would be cut by fifteen percent. They conclude: "Intakes of fat and type of fat were not related to the incidence of the combined outcome of all cardiovascular diseases or to total or cardiovascular mortality."

All this published evidence, of course, does not deter the big pharmaceutical business from coming up with more drugs. Soon doctors will be recommending one pill to lower your LDL level, and another drug to raise your HDL level and lower your triglycerides. This will not only double the already high cost many people are paying for their current statin drugs, but also greatly increase your risk of suffering a stroke, or dying from cancer or any other disease.

Even aggressive behavior and suicides are now linked with lowering cholesterol levels. Since 1992, researchers have noted increases in suicides among those undertaking cholesterol-lowering treatment or dietary regimes. By lowering blood cholesterol you also reduce serotonin receptors leading to increased micro viscosity and affecting the balance of cerebral lipid metabolism. This is believed to have profound effects on brain function. Data from mental institutions have revealed that aggressive people and those with antisocial personality have lower blood cholesterol levels than average. Mental patients with high blood cholesterol levels were found to be less regressed and withdrawn than those with lower levels.

After so many years of researching heart disease and its risk factors, there is no evidence to date linking high cholesterol levels to heart disease, stroke or any other disease as a cause-and-effect relationship, although in some cases both may occur together. The decision to embark on lifelong cholesterol lowering drug treatment in patients with primary hypercholesterolemia depends on the doctor's interpretation of available evidence. However, such evidence exists only for those who have a vested interest in keeping the cholesterol myth alive. At the same time, the true culprits or contributing factors of vascular diseases remain largely concealed from the public's eye. Yet it is becoming increasingly evident that a diet high in animal proteins poses, perhaps, the greatest physical risk for arterial damage and subsequent buildup of cholesterol-containing plaque.

Cholesterol – Your Life and Blood

A newborn baby that is being breast-fed by its mother receives a high dose of cholesterol right from the beginning of its life. Mother's milk contains twice the cholesterol of cow's milk! Nature certainly has no intention of destroying a baby's heart by giving it such high amounts of cholesterol. On the contrary, a healthy heart consists of 10% pure cholesterol (all water removed). Our brain is made of even more cholesterol than the heart is and half of our adrenal glands consist of it. Cholesterol is an essential building block of all our body cells and is needed for every metabolic process. Because cholesterol is such an important substance for the body every single cell is capable of producing it. We could not even live a single day without it.

Cholesterol

- is important for brain development
- protects the nerves against damage or injury
- repairs damaged arteries (seals off lesions)
- supports immune functions
- gives elasticity to red blood cells
- stabilizes and protects cell membranes
- is the basic ingredient of most sexual hormones
- helps to form the skin
- is the essential substance which the skin uses to make vitamin D
- is the basic ingredient used to manufacture the body's stress hormones
- is needed to form bile acids to help digestion of fats and keep us lean
- helps to prevent kidney damage in diabetes

Cholesterol plays a vital role in every living being. Microbes, bacteria, viruses, plants, animals, and human beings all depend on it. Since cholesterol is so important for our body, we cannot solely depend on its supply from external sources, but must be able to produce it independently as well. Normally, our body makes about half a gram to one gram of cholesterol a day, depending on how much the body requires at the time. The main cholesterol producers are the liver and the small intestines. These organs release the cholesterol into the blood stream where it is instantly tied to blood proteins that are responsible for transporting it to their designated areas for the purposes listed above. Cholesterol consists of fat and protein molecules, which gives it the name "Lipo Protein." Only about five percent of our cholesterol circulates in the blood, the rest is used for numerous activities in the body's cells.

If a healthy person consumed 100g of butter a day (the average European eats 18g a day), he would ingest 240-mg cholesterol, of which only 30-60% would be absorbed through his intestines. This would give him about 90 mg cholesterol each day. Yet of this amount, only 12 mg would eventually end up in his blood and raise the cholesterol level by as little as 0.2%. In comparison, our body is able to produce 400 times more cholesterol than we could obtain from eating 100g butter. In other words, if you eat more than the usual amount of cholesterol with your food, your blood cholesterol levels will naturally rise. However, to balance this increase your body will automatically reduce its own cholesterol production. This self-regulating mechanism ensures that cholesterol remains on the exact level that your body requires in order to sustain optimal functions and equilibrium.

If eating fatty foods does not significantly increase cholesterol levels to meet the body's demands for this vital substance then the body must take other more drastic measures. One of them is the stress response. If your body runs low in cholesterol, you are likely to feel stressed. You will loose your calm and patience, and feel tense. Stress is a powerful trigger for cholesterol production in the body. Since cholesterol is the basic constituent of all stress hormones, any unsettling situation will use up large quantities of cholesterol. To make up for the loss or increased demand of cholesterol, the liver starts making more of it.

Take the example of the cholesterol-increasing effect of television. Research has shown that watching television for several hours at a time can drive up blood cholesterol more dramatically than any other so called risk factors, including diet, sedentary lifestyle, or genetic disposition. Exposure to television is a great challenge for the brain. It is far beyond it's the brain's capacity to process the flood of incoming stimuli that emanate from the overwhelming number of picture frames appearing on the TV screen every second. The resulting strain takes its toll. Blood pressure rises to help move more oxygen, glucose, cholesterol, vitamins, and other nutrients around the body and to the brain, all of which are used up rapidly by the heavy brainwork. Add violence, suspense and the noise of gunshots etc., to the spectacle and the adrenal glands respond with shots of adrenaline to prepare the body for a "fight or flight". This causes contraction of many large and small blood vessels in the body, leading to shortage of water, sugar and other nutrients in the cells.

The signs for this stress-response can be several. You may feel shattered, exhausted, and stiff in neck and shoulders, very thirsty, lethargic, depressed, and even "too tired" to go to sleep. If the body did not bother to increase cholesterol levels during such stress encounters, we would have millions of television deaths by now. Thanks to rising cholesterol levels!

When Cholesterol Signals SOS

The self-regulating cholesterol mechanism that keeps the body healthy even in stressful situations is disrupted when the body has begun to store excessive amounts of protein in the liver capillaries. The liver capillaries, called *sinusoids*, are grid-shaped, and their thin basal membranes have sizable pores that normally permit larger molecules and even the relatively large blood cells to leave the blood stream and enter the fluids surrounding liver cells. Unlike other cells, liver cells are thus able to work directly with the blood and its contents.

In comparison with the High Density Lipoprotein (HDL), also known as "good" cholesterol, the Low Density Lipoprotein (LDL) as well as Very Low Density Lipoprotein (VLDL), termed "bad" cholesterol, are relatively large cholesterol molecules. Despite their size, the latter two are still able to pass through the sinusoids and enter the liver cells where they are rebuilt, sent to the gallbladder for storage, or excreted into the intestines. In fact, most of these large cholesterol molecules cannot "escape" the blood stream anywhere else, but through the liver sinusoids. Only the small HDL molecules, which make up 80% of all lipoproteins, are small enough to pass through ordinary capillaries in different parts of the body. For this reason, HDL is hardly ever found to reach abnormally high levels in the blood. LDL and VLDL, on the other hand, may rise to levels that reflect an underlying disorder (congestion) of some sort.

Under normal circumstances, most of the cholesterol eaten in a meal is absorbed by the small intestine and sent to the liver. Once the larger LDL and VLDL molecules enter the liver they are removed from the blood in the manner described before. This mechanism, which keeps the cholesterol concentration of the blood balanced, becomes defective when the normal outlets for cholesterol, namely the grid fibers of the sinusoids, become blocked by excessive amounts of stored proteins. Consequently LDL and VLDL concentrations begin to rise in the blood to levels that indicate the occurrence of blockage and, possibly, inflammatory processes in the sinusoids and coronary arteries. The "bad" cholesterol is trapped in the circulatory system because its escape routes, the liver sinusoids, are congested. The liver's sinusoids become congested with proteins whenever the capillary and artery walls in the rest of the body are congested. The injuries caused by the proteins require much of the bad cholesterol to be used as a band-aid to prevent possible occurrences of heart attack. Eventually, however, the arteries become increasingly hard, rigid, and occluded. This may raise arterial blood pressure and pose further problems to the heart.

The vicious cycle closes when the liver cells are no longer able to receive enough of the LDL and VLDL cholesterol. They naturally assume that the blood does not contain sufficient amounts of cholesterol. The liver cells subsequently begin to produce extra quantities of cholesterol which they pass into the bile ducts. Much of the cholesterol intermixes with bile and is then dispatched to the intestines where it combines with fats and enters the blood stream. This may raise the blood cholesterol levels even further. Some of the affected individuals produce twice as much LDL as a healthy person does.

In the presence of toxic substances and due to lack of bile salts some of the excessive cholesterol forms intrahepatic stones (consisting of mostly cholesterol). These stones decrease bile flow and further reduce the body's ability to digest protein and fat-containing foods. Every meal that contains cholesterol – a natural part of numerous foods – adds more of the "bad" cholesterol to the one that is already trapped in the blood stream. The body's final attempt to stay alive is to accommodate more and more cholesterol in the bile ducts and tissue of the liver, which could end up leading to an enlarged, fatty liver, and to stick as much cholesterol as possible to the damaged walls of the arteries.

In many cases, the liver's sinusoids become so congested with proteins that they do not even allow enough water and sugar to reach the liver cells. As a result, many of the liver cells simply die off. The dead liver cells are replaced with fibrous tissue, leading to portal hypertension, diabetes, and possibly liver failure. And because the protein storage does not only occur in the liver sinusoids, but also in the capillaries and arteries throughout the body, the risk of a heart attack or stroke increases dramatically.

Cholesterol cannot be considered a culprit for heart disease or any other illness. Due to protein deposits in the sinusoids the liver cells are increasingly cut off from the daily needed cholesterol supplies, and are therefore forced to synthesize more and more cholesterol. Lowering blood cholesterol by cutting out fats in the diet and/or artificially reducing it through statin drugs has little or no benefits in the control of heart disease. What helps most is cutting out all animal protein (meat, fish, poultry, eggs, cheese, milk) from the diet plan, until the condition has been completely normalized. If any of these foods are being reintroduced, they should only be eaten occasionally and very sparingly. At the same time, all gallstones in the liver bile ducts and gallbladder should be removed through a series of liver cleanses, and the colon should be cleansed from any existing waste deposits. Additional essential measures include drinking plenty of water (6-8 glasses per day), maintaining a healthy diet and lifestyle, and, if necessary, giving blood to reduce excessive amounts of protein from the blood and to lower the Hemocrit value. All this can effectively reverse atherosclerosis and prevent a heart attack or stroke.

Balancing Cholesterol Naturally

Apart from the above methods, there a number of herbal substances and foods that have powerful cleansing effects on the blood vessels and lymphatic ducts. When ingested regularly, they naturally balance blood cholesterol concentrations to where they need to be for the body to function optimally. Take for example, the extract from a common Indian tree known as the *mukul myrrh* or *guggul.* Guggul is no strange medicine in India. Ayurvedic doctors have used it for over 3,000 years to treat a variety of diseases. One side benefit happens to be the lowering of cholesterol and triglycerides. Double blind clinical trials in India have proven that the extract of this small thorny tree is just as effective for this as some common prescription drugs. Of course, what heals common ailments naturally is unattractive to big drug companies, and, therefore, stands no chance of making it into the field of mainstream medicine, at least not in countries where the pharmaceutical giants dominate health care.

There are dozens of herbs and common foods that all have similar effects as guggul. Green tea alone has shown to have great benefits for cholesterol health. Most fruits and vegetables, including apples, citrus fruit, berries, carrots, apricots, cabbage, and sweet potatoes have also shown to be helpful in naturally balancing cholesterol. Almonds walnuts, pumpkin seeds, olive oil, coconut oil, oats, barley, etc., are just as effective.

Recently, the drug giants declared war on red yeast rice, and succeeded banning it in the U.S. Several studies show that this ancient Asian edible slashed cholesterol an average of 40 points in just 3 months, without any side effects whatsoever. As its reputation increased, it became a serious threat to the greatest drug-sellers of all time – statins. To secure the continuance of the big business, red yeast rice needed to be eliminated, thanks to the FDA.

Lemon rind and orange peel contain a substance that lowers cholesterol quite dramatically. Even the researchers were shocked when they tested *policosanol*—a safe, natural substance found in citrus peels. In one study, 244 women with high cholesterol received either a placebo or policosanol. Researchers saw the bad cholesterol of the policosanol group plunge by 25%. Total cholesterol fell 17%. In addition, their ratio of total to good cholesterol (*the* most important risk factor) *improved* by a whopping 27.2%! Another study compared policosanol against a popular statin drug. Those given policosanol lowered their bad cholesterol by an average of 19.3% – versus just 15.6% for the statin. Most important, policosanol improved the most crucial ratio – total cholesterol to good cholesterol – by 24.4% (the statin drug only improved it by 15.9%). Just chewing on organic lemon rind once daily may be enough to balance cholesterol.

Food is still by far the best medicine for most ailments plaguing the human body. If used wisely, and without destroying it before its consumption, food can create miraculous cures of the most common diseases. I have discussed a number of such healing foods and herbs in *Timeless Secrets of Health & Rejuvenation*. When choosing the right healing foods for you, please refer to the food lists shown in that book. Foods that harmonize with one's body type have the most healing properties, whereas foods that do not may actually interfere with the body's own effort to restore health and vitality.

Overcoming Heart Disease –
Two Encouraging Testimonies

Over the course of several decades, I have seen hundreds of patients with "heart" problems that, in fact, were not heart problems at all. Most of these turned out to be cases of simple indigestion, causing strong sensations of pain in the chest and stomach. Their stomachs were usually hard and swollen, filled with pockets of gas exerting great pressure on the diaphragm and heart. Trapped gas and "heart burn" more often than not lead to the false alarm of a heart condition. Other patients, however, did have serious heart trouble, in addition to suffering chronic indigestion, or, as I see it, because of it. George, age 64, was one of them.

George had received medical treatment for thirty years for what his cardiologist called "progressive heart disease." During the same period, he had been on a large variety of drugs to relieve the symptoms. One of them was an anti-hypertensive drug. The drug's diuretic effects helped to drain excess fluids from his body, but also caused severe cellular dehydration and damaged his kidneys and liver. Other side effects included impotence, increase of angina pain, stomach upset, eye pains, muscle weakness, depression, and nightmares.

Despite taking the drugs regularly, he was advised to undergo a bypass operation since several of his heart arteries were almost completely blocked. A few years after the operation, at age 62, his "new" coronary arteries also showed strong signs of damage, causing chest pain and severe tiredness. His heart was no longer able to perform sufficiently well and, he was informed that, as a last resort, only a heart replacement could prolong his life. That was the time I saw George for the first time. He said this to me: "I feel more dead than alive. My energy level is only a fraction of what it used to be. There is not much I can do now except wait for a heart replacement, but considering my general condition I am not sure whether I even can make it through such an operation."

After applying the diagnostic tools of Ayurvedic Pulse Reading and Eye Interpretation, I explained to him that his real problem wasn't his heart, but the amassed, and toxic, undigested food in his intestines (I was pointing to his grossly protruded belly), and the stored animal protein throughout his blood vessel system. The toxic material was suffocating the cells of his body and causing slow poisoning of the liver, kidney, and heart cells. His liver bile ducts were congested with thousands of gallstones. I suggested that he remove all the toxic waste, which his body had collected over the past 40 years in his small and large intestines through intestinal cleansing, and stimulate the digestive power through a series of liver cleanses. Thereby, he could directly relieve his heart from the heavy burden of having to deliver nutrients to a body that was blocked and overtaxed with harmful material. His heart was obviously exhausted from pumping blood through a congested body.

George quickly began to implement a program that included directions for a specific body-type diet, cleansing of his intestines and liver, the daily and seasonal Ayurvedic routine, regular full body oil massage, yoga and walking near the beachfront, and meditation.

Within three days of his first-ever colonic irrigation session, and strict avoidance of any protein foods, George felt a huge burden had been lifted from his heart. His energy began to return, but he still did not feel strong enough to go back to work. Two weeks later, though, he was back at his desk, with great enthusiasm. Being a director of his own successful insurance company, he no longer felt as stressed at work as he used to feel before the treatment. He was also asleep by 10 p.m. and meditating each day, which made him feel refreshed and calm, and able to handle the difficulties at work with a more relaxed attitude.

Three months later, George visited his cardiologist who took him through a series of tests to determine the condition of his heart. George was not surprised to hear his doctor confirm that he no longer needed a heart transplant operation. He saved himself the $750,000.00 that the heart transplant would have cost. Over time, he reduced and finally stopped all of his medications. Ten years later, he is still very active and enjoys an excellent state of health.

"Just thought you would like to hear the latest report from my cardiologist, whom I went to see on Monday, just because it has now been over one year since my heart attack." This was the beginning of an e-mail message that Susan, a 62-year old friend of mine from Arizona, sent me in the year 2000. "He was a bit disturbed when I first saw him," she continued, "because I said I was not taking any medications and had not done so since last August. As he was talking with me, he said he would probably prescribe a couple of medications for me to start taking again, but first he wanted to do an echocardiogram and a stress test."

" agreed to them both and they were done in his office. While I was on the treadmill, I became tired, so I told his assistants I was getting tired and they said 'You may be, but your heart is not!' They said the echocardiogram and stress test were well within normal limits. When the cardiologist came back into the room, he said, 'I am totally surprised, just totally surprised. These tests show a healthy heart, no failure at all! So you can go home, continue doing what you have been doing and come back to see me in six months.' He did not mention anything else about medications."

Her message ended by saying how grateful she was for having received all the advice and recommendations that had given her the power to claim a healthy normal heart. Susan is one in thousands of people who were listed as incurable heart disease patients, but through liver cleansing and changes in diet and lifestyle, has beaten the odds.

Non-dietary Causes of Heart Disease

Lack of Social Support System

Traditionally, Japanese people living in Japan have very low rates of heart disease and cancer. But when Japanese began immigrating in large numbers to the United States, their newly adopted lifestyle and diet often proved disastrous for their health. By the second generation in the new world, there was no advantage left with respect to these leading killer diseases. First, it was hypothesized that the typical American diet rich in fats, was responsible for this development. Soon the *heart disease-diet-cholesterol* explanation received a severe blow.

There was one subgroup among the Japanese immigrants in California who continued to have very low rates of heart disease, irrespective of whether their blood cholesterol levels were high or low. The group consisted of males who retained their sense of being Japanese by growing up in a Japanese neighborhood, by participating in traditional Japanese cultural and social events, and by learning and speaking their mother tongue. The close family ties and social support system were the only factors that prevented them from developing degenerative heart disease. Even if they had personal problems at home or financial difficulties, there was a large family to lean on and to receive moral and often financial support.

A Swedish study proved that frequent social interaction among men – friendships, golf outings, poker nights, etc. – correlated into a more than 50% reduction in heart disease among test subjects. As far as I know there is no prescription drug that could boast such results, not even close. The feeling of being rejected, left behind and lonely can be a "heart-breaking" event that easily can turn a healthy heart into a sick heart. Most physicians know that women are in greater need of support and understanding during pregnancy. In fact, an epidemiological study on pregnant women showed that 91 percent of those who felt unsupported by family and friends suffered serious complications during pregnancy. The women reported that they were leading stressful lives with little or no social support. Similar studies on unemployed men have revealed that those men who felt strong support from family, relatives and friends were less likely to develop physical or mental problems.

Greatest Risk Factors:
Job Satisfaction and Happiness Rating

What is rarely mentioned in reports on heart disease and their contributing risk factors is one the most important discoveries ever made about man's number one killer disease: *The greatest risks of developing heart disease are job satisfaction and happiness rating.* These unexpected risk factors turned up when

American researchers looked once more at clues of what could cause heart disease.

If you ask a man in the street whether he is satisfied with his job and happy, depending on his answer, you will be able to make a prognosis about whether he is at risk of developing heart disease or not. It would be too simplistic to assume that heart disease is *only* caused by stress, cigarette smoking, overeating, alcohol abuse, etc. These risk factors are not the ultimate causes of a dysfunctional heart, but rather the effects or symptoms of plain dissatisfaction in life. The cause behind the major causes of heart disease, which is nothing but the plain lack of happiness and contentment in life, may still be there after all the other risk factors or causes have been eliminated. A large number of people have died from heart attacks with perfectly clean arteries and no other tangible, physical reasons. Many of them have never smoked, abused alcohol, or led a particularly stressful life. However, they were unhappy within themselves.

One 1998 study by the Johns Hopkins School of Medicine has confirmed what 10 other surveys have found: Clinically depressed men are twice as likely to suffer heart attacks or develop other heart illnesses as those who are not unhappy or depressed. If the "heartache" is severe enough, there are several ways to shut down the arteries and, in fact, the entire energy system in the body. DNA research has shown that the double strands of the DNA controlling the health of every cell in your body suddenly contract and shorten when you feel fear, frustration, anger, jealously, or hatred. It is as if the software of a computer program begins to malfunction and the computer does no longer perform properly. By applying the procedure of Kinesiology[12] muscling testing to a depressed or unhappy person, you find that all the muscles in his body are weak, especially while he ponders his personal problems. His discontent also affects the muscles of his heart and arteries. If unhappiness persists, disease is inevitable, and whatever part of his body is the weakest will succumb first to the chronic shortage of energy. If it happens to be the heart, then heart disease may result.

Even if such a person doses himself with antioxidants, which are believed to protect the arteries against oxygen radical attacks, they will neither be digested and assimilated, nor be successfully delivered to the damaged arteries. Lack of satisfaction in life paralyzes the body's functions of digestion, metabolism, and elimination. This causes congestion, high toxicity, and damage to all cell tissues. People who have blocked coronary arteries are not just

---

[12] For exact directions, see Chapter 1 of *Timeless Secrets of Health and Rejuvenation.*

sick in the area of the heart, they are sick throughout the body. The most important determinant factor of disease appears to be the inability to live a happy, satisfying life.

The reason modern medicine is so helpless in providing lasting cures of heart disease is that there is not much in the current medical approach that can increase happiness in a patient. Yet there is hardly any other primary risk factor for disease, including coronary heart disease, other than its absence. It is the lack of lasting happiness and peace of heart and mind that makes a person feel stressed, take drugs, overeat protein and other foods, abuse alcohol and cigarettes, drink excessive amounts of coffee, become a workaholic, or dislike his job or himself.

Your Need to Love

Satisfaction in life increases spontaneously when we devote time to meet our spiritual needs, apart from developing our physical and mental aspects. The human self cries out to be recognized as a spiritual being whose innate nature is unconditional happiness. A truly happy person finds deep inner satisfaction in sharing whatever he likes about himself with others; this is called love. Love is the most basic characteristic of a human being. Love is the life force that makes the heart beat, the cells thrive, and the spirit sore. However, at times it becomes overshadowed or remains unexpressed. If it is unable to flow inside and outside the body, it causes deep sadness and frustration in the heart center.

Having a doctor identify a few risks of disease and "treating them away" does nothing for a person's profound inner need to open his heart to others and to himself. Such an approach is futile because it ignores the fact that human feelings are far more powerful than any physical effect could ever be. If unhappiness continues to prevail in a patient's life, no amount of vitamin C or E will stop free radicals from creating havoc in the body.

The continual emphasis on the risk factors for disease today may divert people's attention from the real issues in life. That happiness rating and job satisfaction are the leading causes of heart disease is hardly being publicized because there doesn't seem to be a magic formula to deal with them. The pharmaceutical industry possesses no drugs that can make people happy; all it can offer is drugs that deal with the physical symptoms of the disease. If you are troubled with heart disease, you may need to ask yourself a few basic questions, such as these:

Am I living a lifestyle that is detrimental to my health, and if yes, why would I do that? Do I feel that no one really likes or loves me? Am I afraid of being rejected by my partner? Do I believe that I have a deeper purpose in my life, but cannot find it? Am I feeling frustrated because I am not able to get out of life what I really want? Most importantly, am I afraid to love, out of fear of becoming hurt?

The Power of A Loving Spouse

Major research on male heart attack patients has shown that the men's feeling of being loved by their wives was the most crucial element that determined whether they survived an attack or not. Heart attacks often turn into a revelation for estranged couples who have forgotten how to love and care about each other. The sudden closeness which couples often experience after one partner suffers a heart attack can serve as an incentive for many of the patients to continue wanting to live, and the chances are that they *will* live.

Surveys of male heart attack victims revealed that most men felt lonely or misunderstood before their attack. Minor attacks led to death only in those men who felt that their spouse no longer loved them. If a relationship was brought back to "life" because of the attack, then even a massive heart attack could not take the person's life. Most men are quite sensitive at heart, even though they may not necessarily admit it. They generally tend to put on a brave face and suffer silently when they have "heartache." Most men tend to consider it a sign of weakness to shed tears, especially if it is in front of a woman. Yet the male's tendency to repress feelings of weakness makes him a likely candidate for heart disease. A heart attack can reveal his deep vulnerability and yearning for support and comfort. He allows his partner to see this "new" side of him, which can trigger love, compassion, a new sense of intimacy, and give a new lease on life to both of them.

A new European study, from the U.K., confirmed all the earlier findings. It showed that having loving, close relationships – with spouses, relatives or close friends – helped to measurably lower heart attack victims' risk of suffering a second cardiovascular event. In fact, heart attack survivors that do not have an intimate relationship to lean on for emotional support or social interaction are twice as likely to suffer major heart problems within one year of their initial heart attack.

The Healing Power of "Loving Touch"

Every time someone touches us with loving care or we do the same for someone else, an emotional exchange takes place that profoundly nourishes the heart. The expressions "He touched my heart", "I felt so touched by his words," or "It was so touching to see my old friend again", show that the sense of touch is closely related to our physical and emotional heart, which is also the center of our being. To touch and to be touched is as essential to health as a balanced diet, if not more.

When American researchers discovered that prematurely born babies who are stroked three times a day increased their weight by 49 percent, they had unintentionally discovered the *loving touch*. As it turned out, loving touch – the scientific expression is *kinesthetic tactile stimulation* - became recognized as an effective method to reduce the time and cost of a baby's stay in hospital. Loving touch (I prefer to use the less sterile and more human term for this precious gift of God) stimulated the babies' production of growth hormones and thereby improved utilization of nutrients from the daily food ratio. The researchers did not realize that they had stumbled upon a major technique of healing that could be applied successfully to the young and the old, the healthy and the sick, and not only for prevention, but also for cure.

In the human body, the sense of touch is so highly developed that it can detect or sense everything it comes into contact with, like radar. By (unconsciously) picking up other people's *pheromones*[13] and/or "touching" their aura, your body can identify who is friendly, honest and loving or cold-hearted, deceitful, and aggressive. The body may instantly translate all that information into powerful chemical responses that can make you either feel well or ill. These internal responses, however, also depend on your interpretation of the experience. Muscle testing can verify whether your interpretation is correct. You may think of a person and check with your muscles whether this person has a positive influence on you or not. A weak muscle indicates that your relationship with this person may disturb your balance and energy field. Merely thinking of a person gives you enough physical responses to decide whether you want to be with that person or not.

---

[13]   Chemicals produced by the body that signals its presence to others. Pheromones play a particularly important role in sexual behavior. It has become crystal clear that human pheromones affect us more than most people can imagine. Our knowledge of visual input, and of how vision might influence our sexual behavior, pales by comparison.

There are multiple forms of touch that can have profound healing effects. The Ayurvedic oil massage, for example, has been proven to open clogged arteries because of its deeply penetrating and detoxifying action. However, the purely physical part of this kind of touch is only partly responsible for this healing phenomenon. By touching your body with the intention to improve its health, it automatically senses that you love and appreciate yourself and your life; otherwise, you would not do it. Love carries the highest frequency of energy, and, when present in the depth of your heart, it triggers a strong healing response by releasing *endorphins*[14] and other healing drugs throughout the body, similar to the ones a breast-fed baby receives from its mother.

If you want to help a sick person, but do not know how, hold his/her hand in yours, or gently hold or massage his/her feet. This does more to help the person's condition than any amount of sympathetic words could do. The body remembers a loving touch more vividly than spoken words and it reproduces the same drugs whenever it links into the "touching" feeling through remembering. Heart patients especially need to feel that they are loved and cared for because their hearts have lost the

---

[14]   Endorphins are hormones produced by the body that stop pain and make you feel good (pleasure drugs).

sweetness of life that is mostly present in a committed and loving relationship where emotional exchange is most common. Many heart disease victims have isolated themselves from such intimacy before they became ill, by overloading themselves with work, commitments, deadlines, and too many social engagements. By rediscovering the secrets of loving touch, they can once again connect to the circuit of love that supplies the only frequency the heart needs in order to function properly and efficiently, that is, the love frequency.

Loving touch opens the heart. It is the kind of touch that gives without expecting anything in return. It is the kind of touch that can create miracles. Each one of us has this healing gift; it is only a matter of acknowledging that you have it, which is a prerequisite for being able to use it. Give your touch freely and without reservations, for it is one of the few gifts that can make you truly happy, too. It may feel nice to be loved by someone, but it is most important to express love to others, in whatever form is possible. You always have the choice to touch someone with your kindness, generosity, and honesty, and feel so much better for it. This opens your heart. Only a closed heart can be broken or attacked.

Living your whole life without the danger of suffering a heart attack is more your choice

108

than something that just happens to you. Take care of your heart and it will take care of you.

Conclusion:

The modern heart disease epidemic merely reflects the enormous transition we are passing through on an emotional, physical and spiritual level at this crucial time in human history. We have collectively created this epidemic to deal with our emotions and to turn the planet of fear into a planet of love. Since emotions are mental impulses that have physical expressions we can effectively balance them by clearing any obstructions that may have occurred in the heart, the blood and lymph vessels, the liver, kidneys, intestines and other organs.

Heart disease is not difficult to reverse. However, since heart disease indicates that all elements of body, mind and spirit are struggling with dis-ease, all of them must be made whole and healthy again. What becomes more and more clear in our search for health is that we need to take recourse to simple solutions to tackle complex health problems. These solutions are available to those take active self-responsibility for their health and well being. The desire to mend the heart or any other sick part of the body through non-invasive, non-violent and natural means is an impulse of love that opens the heart. It also opens the door to recognizing Spirit within.

Removing gallstones from the liver and gallbladder can by itself prevent and reverse heart disease especially if it is combined with programs of hydration and improved diet/lifestyle. A clean liver is perfectly capable of protecting the heart and its blood vessels from becoming blocked and damaged. If heart disease has already occurred, other organs such as the kidneys and intestines must be cleansed, too. The lymphatic system, which serves as the body's waste removal system, has to be clear of any congestion for the body's cells to enjoy stress-free and frictionless functioning.

Cleansing does not only free your cells from struggle and strive, but also liberate you on all levels. It is good to remind ourselves that whatever we do on the physical planes we automatically do on the emotional and mental planes as well. In addition to restoring balance in our body, we spontaneously restore balance in our world. Although heart disease can be a devastating experience for a person and his loved ones, it can also be an opportunity for a quantum leap in personal development.

Useful Tips to Reverse Heart Disease[15]

To effectively remove congestion in the body and reverse heart disease and hypertension you need to do the following things:

- Remove gallstones from the liver and gallbladder through a series of liver flushes combined with colon cleanses.
- Dissolve kidney stones or sand through kidney cleansing.
- Drink a minimum of six to eight glasses of water a day,
- Avoid iced beverages and drinking with meals.
- Take the main meal of the day at around midday, and the lightest meal in the evening before 7 p.m.
- Go to sleep before 10 p.m.
- Exercise for a minimum of 10-15 minutes a day.
- Reduce or cut out these protein foods: meat, fish, pork, poultry, eggs, cheese, milk, soy, power drinks).
- Avoid stimulants that act as diuretics (tea, coffee, cigarettes, sodas, alcoholic beverages).

---

[15] For detailed information and explanations, refer to the author's books *The Amazing Liver & Gallbladder Flush* and *Timeless Secrets of Health & Rejuvenation.*

111

- Avoid commercial table salt, but include natural sea salt or rock salt in your diet.
- To remove accumulated waste matter from the tissues, the lymphatic system and the blood, take 1-2 sips of hot, ionized water (boiled for 15 minutes and kept in a thermos) every half hour throughout the day, for several weeks.
- Set aside time for meditation and recreation every day.
- Remove heavy metals, chemicals, pesticides, herbicides, absorbed plastics and toxins through *"Natural Cellular Defense"* (order through this website http://www.mywaiora.com/390340).
- To keep the body's mineral composition in balance, use liquid ionic minerals as found in VIBE by Eniva 866-999-9191 or 763-398-0005 (you may use the author's ordering ID13462), or visit this web site: https://enivamembers.com/enerchi
- To maintain healthy cell membranes, strengthen the immune system and support optimal heart health, use *Ambrotose complex* and *CardioBalance* by Mannatech. Visit http://www.mannapages.com/andreasmoritz

ABOUT THE AUTHOR

Andreas Moritz is a medical intuitive, a practitioner of Ayurveda, Iridology, Shiatsu and Vibrational Medicine, a writer and artist. Born in Southwest Germany in 1954, Andreas had to deal with several severe illnesses from an early age, which compelled him to study diet, nutrition and various methods of natural healing while still a child.

By the age of 20, Andreas had completed his training in Iridology – the diagnostic science of eye interpretation – and Dietetics. In 1981, he began studying Ayurvedic Medicine in India and completed his training as a qualified practitioner of Ayurveda in New Zealand in 1991. Rather than being satisfied with merely treating the symptoms of illness, Andreas has dedicated his life's work to understanding and treating the root causes of illness. Because of this holistic approach, he has had astounding success with cases of terminal disease where conventional methods of healing proved futile.

Since 1988, he has been practicing the Japanese healing art of Shiatsu, which has given him profound insights into the energy system of the body. In addition, he devoted eight years of active research into consciousness and its important role in the field of mind/body medicine.

Andreas Moritz is the author of *The Amazing Liver & Gallbladder Flush, Timeless Secrets of Health and Rejuvenation, Lifting the Veil of Duality, Cancer is Not a Disease, It's Time to Come Alive,*
The Art of Self-Healing (mid-2006), and *Simple Steps to Total Health* (mid-2006).

During his extensive travels throughout the world, he has consulted with heads of state and members of government in Europe, Asia, and Africa, and has lectured widely on the subject of health, mind/body medicine and spirituality. His popular *Timeless Secrets of Health and Rejuvenation* workshops assist people in taking responsibility for their own health and well-being. Andreas runs a free forum "Ask Andreas Moritz" on the popular health website Curezone.com (5 million readers and increasing).

After taking up residency in the United States in 1998, Andreas has been involved in developing a new innovative system of healing – *Ener-Chi Art* – which targets the root causes of many chronic illnesses. Ener-Chi Art consists of a series of light ray-encoded oil paintings that can instantly restore vital energy flow (Chi) in the organs and systems of the body.

Andreas is also the founder of *Sacred Santèmony – Divine Chanting for Every Occasion,* a powerful system of specially

114

generated sound frequencies that can transform deep-seated fears, allergies, traumas and mental/emotional blocks into useful opportunities of growth and inspiration within a matter of moments. Andreas's latest system "Art of Self-Healing" (as Book/CD or DVD), to be released during 2006, is comprised of his Ener-chi Art and specific Sacred Santémony sounds.

Other Books, Products and Services By The Author

The Amazing
Liver & Gallbladder Flush
A Powerful Do It Yourself Tool to Optimize your Health and Wellbeing

In this revised edition of his best selling book, *The Amazing Liver Cleanse,* Andreas Moritz addresses the most common but rarely recognized cause of illness – gallstones congesting the liver. Twenty million Americans suffer from attacks of gallstones every year. In many cases, treatment merely consists of removing the gallbladder, at the cost of $5 billion a year. However, this purely symptom-oriented approach does not eliminate the cause of the illness, and in many cases, sets the stage for even more serious conditions. Most adults living in the industrialized world, and especially those suffering a chronic illness such as heart disease, arthritis, MS, cancer, or diabetes, have hundreds if not thousands of gallstones (mainly clumps of hardened bile) blocking the bile ducts of their liver.

This book provides a thorough understanding of what causes gallstones in the liver and gallbladder and why these stones can be held responsible for the most common diseases so prevalent in the world today. It provides the reader with the knowledge needed to recognize the stones and gives the necessary, do-it-yourself instructions to painlessly remove them in the comfort of one's home. It also gives practical guidelines on how to prevent new gallstones from being formed. The widespread success of *The Amazing Liver & Gallbladder Flush* is a testimony to the power and effectiveness of the cleanse itself. The liver cleanse has led to extraordinary improvements in health and wellness among thousands of people who have already given themselves the precious gift of a strong, clean, revitalized liver.

Timeless Secrets of Health & Rejuvenation – **Breakthrough Medicine for the 21st Century** (499 pages)

This book meets the increasing demand for a clear and comprehensive guide that can help make people self-sufficient regarding their health and well-being. It answers some of the most pressing questions of our time: How does illness arise? Who heals, who doesn't? Are we destined to be sick? What causes aging? Is it reversible? What are the major causes of disease and how can we eliminate them?

Topics include: The placebo and the mind/body mystery; the laws of illness and health; the four most common risk factors of disease; digestive disorders and their effects on the rest of the body; wonders of our biological rhythms and how to restore them if disrupted; how to create a life of balance; why to choose a vegetarian diet; cleansing the liver, gallbladder, kidneys and colon; removing allergies; giving up smoking naturally; Using sunlight as medicine; the 'new' causes of heart disease, cancer and AIDS; and antibiotics, blood transfusions, ultrasounds scans, immunization programs under scrutiny.

Timeless Secrets of Health and Rejuvenation sheds light on all the major issues of health care and reveals that most medical treatments, including surgery, blood transfusions, pharmaceutical drugs, etc., are avoidable when certain key functions in the body are restored through the natural methods described in the book. The reader also learns about the potential dangers of medical diagnosis and treatment as well as the reasons vitamin supplements, 'health' foods, light products, 'wholesome' breakfast cereals, diet foods and diet programs may have contributed to the current health crisis rather than helped resolve it. The book includes a complete program of health care, which is primarily based on the ancient medical system of Ayurveda and the vast amount of experience Andreas Moritz has gained in the field of health during the past 30 years.

Lifting the Veil of Duality –
Your Guide to Living Without Judgment

"Do you know that there is a place inside you -- hidden beneath the appearance of thoughts, feelings and emotions – that does not know the difference between good and evil, right and wrong, light and dark? From that place you embrace the opposite values of life as *One*. In this sacred place you are at peace with yourself and at peace with your world."
Andreas Moritz

In *Lifting the Veil of Duality,* Andreas Moritz poignantly exposes the illusion of duality. He outlines a simple way to remove every limitation that you have imposed upon yourself during the course of living duality. You will be prompted to see yourself and the world through a new lens – the lens of clarity, discernment and non-judgment. And you will find out that mistakes, accidents, coincidences, negativity, deception, injustice, wars, crime and terrorism all have a deeper purpose and meaning in the larger scheme of things. So naturally, much of what you will read may conflict with the beliefs you currently hold. Yet you are not asked to change your beliefs or opinions. Instead, you are asked to have *an open mind,* for only an open mind can enjoy freedom from judgment.

Our personal views and worldviews are currently challenged by a crisis of identity. Some are being shattered altogether. The collapse of our current World Order forces humanity to deal with the most basic issues of existence. You can no longer avoid taking responsibility for the things that happen to you. When you *do* accept responsibility, you also empower and heal yourself.

Lifting the Veil of Duality shows you how you create or subdue your ability to fulfill your desires. Furthermore, you will find intriguing explanations about the mystery of time, the truth and illusion of reincarnation, the misleading value of prayer, what makes relationships work and why so often they don't. Find out why injustice is an illusion that has managed to haunt us throughout the ages. Learn about our original separation from the Source of life and what this means with regard to the current waves of instability and fear so many of us are experiencing.

Discover how to identify the angels living amongst us and why we all have light-bodies. You will have the opportunity to find the ultimate God within you and discover why a God seen as separate from yourself keeps you from being in your Divine Power and happiness. In addition, you can find out how to heal yourself at a moment's notice. Read all about the "New Medicine" and the destiny of the old medicine, the old economy, the old religion and the old world.

Cancer is Not a Disease!
It's A Survival Mechanism
Discover Cancer's Hidden Purpose,
Heal its Root Causes,
And Be Healthier Than Ever

In *Cancer Is Not A Disease* Andreas Moritz proves the point that cancer is the physical symptom reflecting our body's final attempt to eliminate specific life-destructive causes. He claims that removing such causes sets the precondition for complete healing of our body, mind and emotions.

This book confronts you with a radically new understanding of cancer – one that outdates the current cancer model. On average, the conventional approaches of killing, cutting or burning cancerous cells offer most patients a remission rate of merely 7%, and the majority of the few survivors are "cured" for just five years or less. The prominent cancer researcher and professor at the University of California (Berkeley), Dr. Hardin Jones, stated: "Patients are as well, or better off, untreated..." Any published success figures in cancer survival statistics are offset by equal or better scores among those not receiving any treatments. More people are killed by the treatments than saved.

Cancer is Not a Disease shows you why regular cancer treatments can be fatal, what actually causes cancer, and how you can remove the obstacles that prevent the body from healing itself. Cancer is not an attempt on your life; to the contrary, cancer is trying to save it. Unless we change our perception of what cancer really is, it will continue to threaten the life of nearly one out of every two people. This book opens a door for those who wish to turn feelings of victimhood into empowerment and self-mastery, and disease into health.

Topics of the book include:

- Reasons that coerce the body to develop cancer cells
- How to identify and remove the causes of cancer

- Why most cancers disappear by themselves, without medical intervention
- Why radiation, chemotherapy and surgery never cure cancer
- Why some people survive cancer despite undergoing dangerously radical treatments
- The roles of fear, frustration, low self-worth and repressed anger in the origination of cancer
- How to turn self-destructive emotions into energies that promote health and vitality
- Spiritual lessons behind cancer

It's Time to Come Alive!
Start Using the Amazing Healing Powers of Your Body, Mind and Spirit Today!

In this book, the author brings to light man's deep inner need for spiritual wisdom in life and helps the reader develop a new sense of reality that is based on love, power and compassion. He describes our relationship with the natural world in detail and discusses how we can harness its tremendous powers for our personal and humanity's benefit. *Time to Come Alive* challenges some of our most commonly held beliefs and offers a way out of the emotional restrictions and physical limitations we have created in our lives.

Topics include: What shapes our Destiny; using the power of intention; secrets of defying the aging process; doubting - the cause of failure; opening the heart; material wealth and spiritual wealth; fatigue – the major cause of stress; methods of emotional transformation; techniques of primordial healing; how to increase health of the five senses; developing spiritual wisdom; the major causes of today's earth changes; entry into the new world; twelve gateways to heaven on earth; and many more.

Art of Self-Healing
Instantly Access The Power
To Heal Your Body, Mind and Emotions!
(Available in December 2005)

At this time of great challenge and confusion in all areas of life – individual, social, national and international – we are also blessed with powerful solutions to our most pressing problems. Something we least expected, art and sound are now emerging to become the leading healing methods of our time.

Art of Self-Healing by bestselling author and health practitioner, Andreas Moritz, is a unique approach that gives a person instant access to his/her own healing powers. The approach consists of a series of 32 light-ray-imbued pictures (Ener-Chi Art) created by the author, and specific healing sounds (Sacred Santémony) that he has recorded on CD for the purpose of removing any obstacles to healing one's body and mind and emotions. The supplied CD is synchronized with viewing the pictures for about half a minute each.

All books are available as paperback copies and electronic books (except Art of Self-Healing) from the Ener-Chi Wellness Center.

Website: http://www.ener-chi.com
Email: Enerchiart@aol.com

Phone: (864) 848 6410 or (615) 676-9961

Sacred Santémony – for Emotional Healing

Sacred Santémony is a unique healing system that uses sounds from specific words to balance deep emotional/spiritual imbalances.

The powerful words produced in Sacred Santémony are made from whole-brain use of the letters of the *ancient language* – language that is comprised of the basic sounds that underlie and bring forth all physical manifestation. The letters of the ancient language vibrate at a much higher level than our modern languages, and when combined to form whole words, they generate feelings of peace and harmony (Santémony) to calm the storms of unrest, violence and turmoil, both internal and external.

In April 2002, I spontaneously began to chant sounds that are meant to improve certain health conditions. These sounds resembled chants by Native Americans, Tibetan monks, Vedic pundits (Sanskrit) and languages from other star systems (not known on planet Earth). Within two weeks, I was able to bring forth sounds that would instantly remove emotional blocks and resistance or aversion to certain situations and people, foods, chemicals, thought forms, beliefs, etc. The following are but a few examples of what Sacred Santémony is able to assist you with:

- Reducing or removing fear that is related to death, disease, the body, foods, harmful chemicals, parents and other people, lack of abundance, impoverishment, phobias, environmental threats, the future and the past, unstable economic trends, political unrest, etc.

- Clearing or reducing a recent or current hurt, disappointment or anger resulting from past emotional trauma or negative experiences in life.
- Cleansing of the *Akashic Records* (a recording of all experiences the soul has gathered throughout all life streams) from persistent fearful elements, including the idea and concept that we are separate from and not one with Spirit, God or our Higher Self.
- Setting the preconditions for you to resolve your karmic issues not through pain and suffering, but through creativity and joy.
- Improving or clearing up allergies and intolerances to foods, chemical substances, pesticides, herbicides, air pollutants, radiation, medical drugs, pharmaceutical byproducts, etc.
- Undoing the psycho-emotional root causes of any chronic illness, including cancer, heart disease, MS, diabetes, arthritis, brain disorders, depression, etc.

- Resolving other difficulties or barriers in life by "converting" them into the useful blessings that they really are.

To arrange for a personal Sacred Santémony session with Andreas Moritz, please follow the same directions as given for Telephone Consultations.
(As of 2006, the fee for a half hour is $85)

Ener-Chi Art

Andreas Moritz has developed a new system of healing and rejuvenation designed to restore the basic life energy (Chi) of an organ or a system in the body within a matter of seconds. Simultaneously, it also helps balance the emotional causes of illness.

Eastern approaches to healing, such as Acupuncture and Shiatsu, are intended to enhance well-being by stimulating and balancing the flow of Chi to the various organs and systems of the body. In a similar manner, the energetics of Ener-Chi Art is designed to restore a balanced flow of Chi throughout the body.

According to most ancient systems of health and healing, the balanced flow of Chi is the key determinant for a healthy body and mind. When Chi flows through the body unhindered, health and vitality are maintained. By contrast, if the flow of Chi is disrupted or reduced, health and vitality tend to decline.

A person can determine the degree to which the flow of Chi is balanced in the body's organs and systems by using a simple muscle testing procedure. To reveal the effectiveness of Ener-Chi Art, it is important to apply this test both before and after viewing each Ener-Chi Art picture.

To allow for easy application of this system, Andreas has created a number of healing paintings that have been "activated" through a unique procedure that imbues each work of art with specific color rays (derived from the higher dimensions). To receive the full benefit of an Ener-Chi Art picture all that is necessary is to look at it for less than a minute. During this time, the flow of Chi within the organ or system becomes fully restored. When applied to all the organs and systems of the body, Ener-Chi Art sets the precondition for the whole body to heal and rejuvenate itself.

Ener-Chi Ionized Stones

Ener-Chi Ionized Stones are stones and crystals that have been energized, activated, and imbued with life force through a special activation process introduced by Andreas Moritz – the founder of Ener-Chi Art.

Stone ionization has not been attempted before because stones and rocks have rarely been considered useful in the field of healing. Yet, stones have the inherent power to hold and release vast amounts of information and energy. Once ionized, they exert a balancing influence on everything with which they come into contact. The ionization of stones may be one of our keys to survival in a world that is experiencing high-level pollution and destruction of its eco-balancing systems.

In the early evolutionary stages of Earth, every particle of matter within the mantle of the planet contained within it the blueprint of the entire planet, just as every cell of our body contains within its DNA structure the blueprint of our entire body. The blueprint information within every particle of matter is still there – it has simply fallen into a dormant state. The ionization process "reawakens" this original blueprint information, and enables the associated energies to be released. In this sense, Ener-Chi Ionized Stones are alive and conscious, and are able to energize, purify and balance any natural substance with which they come into contact.

By placing an Ionized Stone next to a glass of water or plate of food, the water or food becomes energized, thereby increasing digestibility and nutrient absorption. Ionized stones can also be used effectively in conjunction with Ener-Chi Art – simply place an Ionized Stone on the corresponding area of the body while viewing an Ener-Chi Art picture. For more potential uses please check out the web site given below.

Telephone Consultations

For a Personal Telephone Consultation with Andreas Moritz, please

1. Call or send an email with your name, phone number, address, digital picture (if you have one) of your face and any other relevant information to Andreas.

2. Set up an appointment for the length of time you choose to spend with him. A comprehensive consultation lasts 2 hours or more. Shorter consultations deal with all the questions you may have and the information that is relevant to your specific health issue(s).

Fees (2005/06): $85 for 1/2 hour, $170 for one hour, $255 for 1 1/2 hours, and $340 for 2 hours

Note: Shorter consultations deal with all the questions you may have and the information that is relevant to your specific health issue(s). For a comprehensive consultation, (if you have a digital camera) please take a snapshot of your face (preferably without makeup) and email it to Andreas before your appointment with him. This can greatly assist Andreas in assisting you in your quest for better health.

To order Ener-chi Art pictures,
Ionized Stones and other products
please contact:

Ener-Chi Wellness Center, LLC
Web Site: http://www.ener-chi.com
E-mail: enerchiart@aol.com

Phone: (864) 848-6410 (USA)
E-voice: (615) 676-9961 (USA)

CPSIA information can be obtained at www.ICGtesting.com
Printed in the USA
BVOW082343011012

301914BV00001B/2/A

9 780976 794455